WTO AGREEMENTS & PUBLIC HEALTH

A joint study by the WHO and the WTO Secretariat

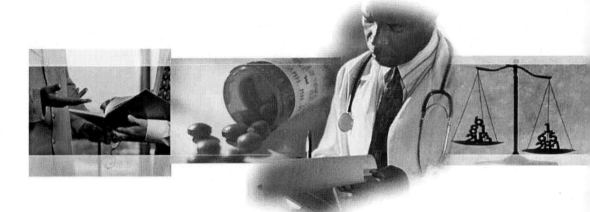

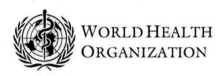

WORLD HEALTH
ORGANIZATION

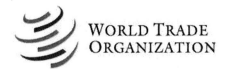

WORLD TRADE
ORGANIZATION

This publication is also available in French and Spanish (Price: SFr 30.-)

WHO ISBN 92 4 156214 5

WTO ISBN 92-870-1223-7

Printed by the WTO Secretariat

VII-2002-6,000

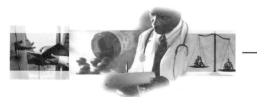

FOREWORD BY
GRO HARLEM BRUNDTLAND AND MIKE MOORE

As the world becomes increasingly integrated, it becomes less and less possible for different policy areas to be handled independently of each other. The linkage between trade and health has been the focus of much debate: real concerns should be dealt with and any misunderstandings should be clarified based on sound evidence and rigorous analysis.

We consider this joint study by the WHO and the WTO Secretariat a useful and timely initiative in this regard. It illustrates that there is much common ground between trade and health. Another important message is that health and trade policymakers can benefit from closer cooperation to ensure coherence between their different areas of responsibilities.

In both the WHO and the WTO questions of trade and public health feature high on the agenda, and significant advances have been made in the recent past. The endorsement by the international community of the Doha Declaration on the TRIPS Agreement and Public Health is a very visible expression of governments' commitment to ensuring that the rules-based trading system is compatible with public health interests.

The multilateral trading system has a lot to contribute to increase global welfare. In addition, the expertise and work of other organizations are needed to find effective solutions. In our common pursuit of sustainable human development, the WTO and the WHO are important partners. We are honoured to present this joint study on WTO Agreements and public health, the first of its kind. It is an encouraging testimony of our good and growing cooperation.

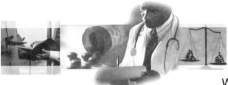

ACKNOWLEDGEMENTS

This report was jointly prepared by the World Health Organization (WHO) and the Secretariat of the World Trade Organization (WTO).

The WHO team was led by Nick Drager and included Robert Beaglehole, Debra Lipson, Zafar Mirza and early input from Matthew Hodge. Information on country health-trade cooperation was kindly provided by Suwit Wibulpolprasert of Thailand's Ministry of Health, and Jake Vellinga of Health Canada. Many WHO staff in Geneva headquarters and six regional offices supplied helpful information and comments at various stages of the report's preparation. We especially thank Orvill Adams, Thiru Balasubramaniam, Douglas Bettcher, William Cocksedge, Sarah England, Julie Milstein, André Prost, Yasuyuki Sahara, Jorgen Schlundt, German Velasquez and Derek Yach for their valuable contributions. WHO's input benefited from the comments of experts around the world, working in government health agencies, academic institutions, and civil society organizations. The WHO team also would like to thank Andrew Cassels, Ann Kern, David Nabarro, Poonam Khetrapal Singh, and Eva Wallstam for their support.

The principal coordinator for the WTO contribution was Deputy Director-General Miguel Rodríguez Mendoza with the assistance of Erik Wijkstrom and Alexander Keck. Inputs and comments were provided by Rolf Adlung, John Finn, David Hartridge, Marion Jansen, Pieter Jan Kuijper, Vivien Liu, João Magelhães, Hamid Mamdouh, Gabrielle Marceau, Doaa Abdel Motaal, Laoise Ni Bhriain, Adrian Otten, Gretchen Stanton, Thu-Lang Tran-Wasescha, Peter Ungphakorn, Jayashree Watal and Frank Wolter. With respect to the WTO, this study has been prepared under the Secretariat's own responsibility and is without prejudice to the positions of WTO Members and to their rights and obligations under the WTO.

The opinions expressed in this report should be attributed to the authors and not to the institutions they represent.

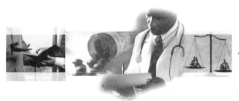

TABLE OF CONTENTS

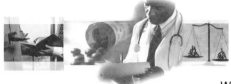

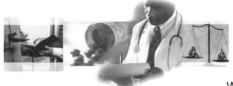

CHARTS AND TABLES

EXECUTIVE SUMMARY

1. This report deals with the relevant WTO Agreements and the way they may influence health and health policies. In undertaking this joint study, the WHO and WTO Secretariats seek to examine the linkages between trade and health policies, so as to enable both trade and health officials to better understand and monitor the effects of these linkages.

The WTO Agreements and public health

2. The first chapter of the report examines the main WTO Agreements related to health and health policies, namely the Agreements on Technical Barriers to Trade (TBT), Sanitary and Phytosanitary Measures (SPS), Trade-Related Intellectual Property Rights (TRIPS), and Trade in Services (GATS). It also refers to the fundamental WTO principles of non-discrimination and national treatment, which guide the actual implementation of the Agreements *inter alia* as they relate to health issues.

3. The basic WTO principle is non-discrimination: WTO Members cannot discriminate between their trading partners nor between imported and locally-produced goods that are otherwise similar. Since the inception of GATT more than 50 years ago, Article XX of GATT guarantees Members' right to take measures to restrict imports and export of products when those measures are necessary to protect the health of humans, animals and plants (Article XX(b)).

4. This and similar provisions in WTO Agreements recognize that there are cases where Members may wish to subordinate trade-related considerations to other legitimate policy objectives and constraints, such as health. WTO jurisprudence, on several occasions, has confirmed that WTO Members have the right to determine the level of health protection they deem appropriate. Human health has been recognized by the WTO as being "important in the highest degree."

5. The above considerations inform the four WTO Agreements examined in this chapter. Both the TBT and SPS Agreements allow countries to restrain trade for legitimate reasons, including health, but they also require that such measures should not unnecessarily restrict trade. Of the two, the SPS Agreement deals with specific risks to health.

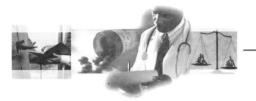

It contains specific rules for countries that want to restrict trade to ensure food safety and the protection of human life from plant- or animal-carried diseases (zoonoses).

6. While the aim of preventing unnecessary trade barriers is common to both the SPS and TBT Agreements, the rights and obligations they entail are somewhat different, for instance with regard to the assessment of health risks. The TBT Agreement has a broader scope of application, but only requires taking available scientific information into account, whereas in the SPS Agreement it is a fundamental requirement that Members have a scientific basis to justify trade measures aimed at mitigating a health risk. If available scientific evidence is not sufficient, the SPS Agreement permits the adoption of provisional measures.

7. The TRIPS Agreement also covers some areas that are relevant to health. The issue of patent protection for pharmaceutical products is particularly critical. This is an area where it is very important to find a proper balance between two complementary public health goals, that of providing incentives for future inventions of new drugs and that of ensuring affordable access to existing drugs.

8. The TRIPS Agreement seeks to help achieving such a balance. It contains several provisions that enable governments to implement their intellectual property regimes in a manner which takes account of immediate and longer-term public health considerations. It also provides for some flexibility in the implementation of the Agreement by allowing countries, under certain conditions, to limit patent owners' exclusive rights, for instance by granting compulsory licenses and allowing parallel importation of patented products. This flexibility was reaffirmed by the WTO Members at the Doha Ministerial Conference.

9. In the case of trade in services, examples relating to health services are given for the four modes of supply. GATS imposes only very limited general obligations on Members, who are free to choose which service sectors to open up and which modes of service to liberalize. Exempt from GATS are any services supplied in the exercise of governmental authority. Market access and national treatment in GATS represent conditional (and negotiable) obligations which may be made subject to conditions or qualifications that Members inscribe in their schedules. This possibility, as well as the continued right to regulate for domestic policy purposes, provide substantial scope for national policy-making, including with regard to health regulations.

The WTO Agreements and some specific health issues

10. While the WTO Agreements explicitly allow governments to take measures to restrict trade in pursuing national health policy objectives, the emphasis in WTO rules is on how policies are pursued without questioning the underlying objective. This chapter looks at the ways in which governments pursue specific health policies and which might have implications for trade. Eight specific health matters are discussed, namely infectious disease control, food safety, tobacco, environment, access to drugs, health services, food security and nutrition, and some emerging issues such as biotechnology. Although the WTO Agreements do not deal directly with all these issues, national policy makers may need to take the Agreements into consideration when addressing them.

Infectious disease control

11. The world today has witnessed the emergence of new global health threats, for which control measures are still evolving (for example HIV/AIDS, Ebola and Marburg viruses). In addition, many "older" diseases (such as tuberculosis, malaria and gonorrhoea) have become a greater threat because they have developed resistance to the drugs commonly used to treat them. In exceptional circumstances, infectious disease control may require trade or travel restrictions, such as quarantines or trade embargoes. Most recently, these have been replaced by a combination of early warning surveillance systems, epidemic preparedness plans, stockpiles of essential medicines, speedy communications, and information sharing through networks, to facilitate quick action.

12. To the extent that trade restrictions are used, they are unlikely to conflict with WTO rules. They are normally time-limited and try to minimize disruption to international trade. This is one of the fundamental principles underlying WHO's International Health Regulations (IHR), which serves as the legal framework for WHO's efforts to prevent disease epidemics from spreading globally. The IHR are in the process of being updated to cope with the new, challenging realities of infectious disease control.

Food Safety

13. Several new sources of food-borne illness are of increasing relevance to international trade (for instance dioxin residues in animal feed or the spread of mad cow dis-

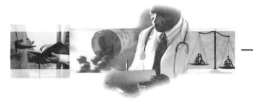

ease (BSE) and its probable onward transmission to people). The trend towards the export of more and more processed foods coupled with growing consumer awareness, and sometimes concern, is increasing the demands relating to safety of traded foods. These issues are covered by the SPS Agreement, which applies to any trade-related measure taken to protect human life or health from risks arising from additives, contaminants, toxins, veterinary drug and pesticide residues, or other disease-causing organisms in foods or beverages.

14. The SPS Agreement clearly gives governments the right to restrict trade to achieve health objectives, but the measures applied must be based on scientific evidence. The SPS Agreement also formally recognizes the food safety standards, guidelines and recommendations established by the FAO/WHO Codex Alimentarius Commission (Codex for short). The WTO beef hormone case underscored the importance of basing food safety regulations on scientific evidence and international food safety standards, but also confirmed the right of Members to have the level of health protection they want, even above international standards. Article 5.7 of the SPS Agreement also authorizes the use of provisional measures when there is a lack of scientific evidence about health risks. The setting of international food safety standards, in particular with regard to new issues such as genetically modified organisms, remains a crucial challenge in the future.

Tobacco control

15. In many countries, governments intervene to reduce tobacco consumption in view of its negative health impacts. While higher tariffs on tobacco contribute to higher consumer prices and lower levels of consumption, governments can use a host of WTO consistent, non-discriminatory measures, such as internal taxes and other tobacco control measures. This is illustrated by the case of Thailand.

16. The challenges to comprehensive tobacco control policies that lie outside national borders led WHO in 1996 to propose the development of a Framework Convention on Tobacco Control (FCTC). Its purpose is to facilitate multilateral cooperation and action at the global level to address transnational tobacco control strategies, for which there is overwhelming empirical evidence as to their effectiveness in reducing demand for tobacco. None of the provisions of the FCTC seem to be inherently WTO-inconsistent; and many of the restrictions called for by some of its provisions may well be determined to be "necessary" for health protection under WTO rules. However, the relationship

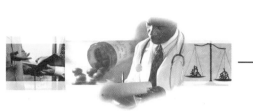

between WTO rules and the FCTC will depend on the direction taken by future negotiations on the FCTC, and the manner in which its rules are applied by governments.

Environment

17. The link between the environment, health and trade is a complex one. Removing trade barriers to modern "green" technologies and to suppliers of environmental goods and services can potentially benefit both the environment and health. For example, the removal of subsidies to polluting industries or to the energy and agricultural sectors could benefit both the environment and associated occupational health. Such efforts constitute a "win-win" situation for both trade and health advocates. However, trade in dangerous materials, such as hazardous wastes and unsafe chemicals, may also increase environmental and occupational health hazards, especially in developing countries, if appropriate handling or disposal cannot be guaranteed. Appropriate environmental policies remain essential. From the point of view of developing countries, where poverty is a major concern and an important obstacle to environmental protection, the opening up of world markets to their exports can be part of the solution. Trade liberalization for developing country exports, along with financial and technology transfers, may help developing countries generate resources to protect the environment and work towards sustainable development.

18. Although the environment *per se* is not a WTO issue, several WTO Agreements and rules are relevant to environmental issues. There have been several environmental-related WTO disputes often centring on the issue of "like product". In making a determination of "likeness", WTO rules permit health risks to be taken into account. In a recent case on asbestos, the Appellate Body found the objective pursued, i.e. the preservation of human life and health, to be "both vital and important in the highest degree", and concluded that an import ban on asbestos was a "necessary" measure to protect human health.

19. Another important issue in this area is the relationship between WTO provisions and trade measures applied pursuant to multilateral environment agreements (MEAs). MEAs represent an important multilateral course of action to address specific environmental issues which may also be relevant to health, such as, for example, limiting the use of ozone-depleting substances. Although no disputes have thus far come to the WTO regarding the trade provisions contained in any MEA, there is scope for both controversy

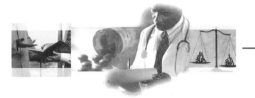

and synergy. There are some 200 MEAs, of which at least 20 contain trade provisions. Some of them may violate the principle of non-discrimination, as they allow for trade with some countries but not with others in like products (a violation of the most-favoured-nation principle), or for discrimination between like domestic and imported products (a violation of the national treatment principle). In the context of the Doha negotiations, countries will be looking more closely at the relationship between existing WTO rules and specific trade obligations set out in MEAs. Members will also be looking at, *inter alia*, procedures for regular information exchange between MEA Secretariats and the relevant WTO committees.

Access to drugs and vaccines

20. WHO estimates that currently one third of the world's population lacks access to essential drugs, and that over 50 per cent of people in poor countries in Africa and Asia do not have access to even the most basic essential drugs. Access to essential medicines and vaccines depends on four critical elements: rational selection and use, sustainable financing, reliable supply systems and affordable prices.

21. Drug prices may be influenced by some WTO Agreements. For example, as WTO negotiations lead to the elimination or reduction of import duties on drugs, vaccines or other medical supplies, this may lower prices. While the TRIPS Agreement should enhance incentives for R & D into new drugs, there is also concern that it may lead to drug price increases due to more stringent patent protection. In this regard, the TRIPS Agreement allows WTO Members, under certain circumstances, to use safeguards, such as compulsory licensing and parallel imports. Although there were some conflicting views regarding the conditions under which the flexibility of the TRIPS Agreement could be used, the Doha Declaration on the TRIPS Agreement and Public Health helps clarify this issue. The Declaration was seen as an important to step to prevent situations where countries have considered themselves under pressure, from industry and/or for-eign governments, not to avail themselves fully of the flexibility provided in the TRIPS Agreement.

22. There is also a range of public policy measures outside the field of intellectual property to address issues of drug prices and access to drugs. Where patent protection confers pricing power for drugs of vital public health or life-saving importance, differen-tial pricing is one way of ensuring that prices in poor developing countries are as low as

possible while higher prices in rich countries continue to provide incentives for R&D. The TRIPS Agreement does not stand in the way of such arrangements.

23. Two cases relevant to the use of the flexibility in the TRIPS Agreement have arisen in the WTO so far. One was a dispute between Canada and the European Communities on the so-called "Bolar" exception allowing generic drug manufacturers to produce and/or import and use quantities necessary of a patented product to conduct tests needed to obtain regulatory approval before the expiry of a patent.

24. The other case was a dispute brought by the United States about the TRIPS consistency of the Brazilian legal framework for the grant of compulsory licences. The United States argued that this provision for the grant of compulsory licenses in the event that a patented invention was not used in domestic production ("local working" requirement) was a protective industrial policy measure and inconsistent with the provisions of the TRIPS Agreement. The Brazilians took the view that this measure was a necessary part of their programme to combat HIV/AIDS and was fully consistent with the TRIPS Agreement. Following bilateral consultations, in July 2001 Brazil and the United States announced that they had reached an understanding and decided to stop their WTO case.

25. Another case concerning access to drugs - not a WTO dispute - that attracted much attention was the challenge in the South African courts by 39 pharmaceutical companies to the South African Medicines and Related Substances Control Amendment Act of 1997. The companies contended that this legislation, which empowered the Minister of Health to authorize and prescribe conditions for the parallel importation of drugs under patent in South Africa, entailed, among other things, a violation of South Africa's obligations under TRIPS. The government argued that its legislation was entirely consistent with the TRIPS Agreement which contains important flexibilities, for instance with regard to parallel importation. No case was brought to the WTO on the grounds that South Africa had breached the TRIPS Agreement. In April 2001, the pharmaceutical companies withdrew their suit, and the South African government pursued the implementation of its regulations, including some that would authorize parallel importation of patented medicines.

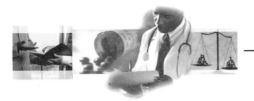

Health services

26. International trade in health services is growing in many areas. Health professionals are moving to other countries, whether on a temporary or permanent basis, usually in search of higher wages and better working conditions. There have also been notable increases in foreign investment by hospital operators and health insurance companies in search of new markets. In addition, more and more countries are seeking to attract health consumers from other countries.

27. Depending on appropriate regulatory conditions, trade liberalization can contribute to enhancing quality and efficiency of supplies and/or increasing foreign exchange earnings. For example, hospitals financed by foreign investors can provide certain services not previously available. In a few developing countries, such as Thailand and Jordan, the health sector serves as a regional supply centre that attracts foreign patients who can contribute to domestic income and employment. Some developing countries, notably Cuba, India and the Philippines, "export" their doctors and nurses, producing foreign exchange remittances and filling supply gaps in host countries.

28. However, not all countries may be well positioned to turn these gains into health benefits for the majority of people. Trade in health services, in some cases, has exacerbated existing problems of access and equity of health services and financing, especially for poor people in developing countries. For example, an increase in the "brain-drain" of health professionals leaving low-income countries to work in higher-income countries can worsen health personnel shortages in developing countries. There are also fears that the benefits of opening markets will be concentrated among the wealthy.

29. Such problems could be addressed through appropriate regulation. GATS leaves countries the flexibility to manage trade in services in ways that are consistent with their national health policy objectives. It is even possible under GATS to impose additional or more rigid requirements on foreign services providers. Trade liberalization heightens the need for effective regulatory frameworks to ensure that private sector activity in the health system generates the expected benefits. While regulatory strategies could be used to reduce unwanted developments, enforcement capacity may be weak in some countries.

30. The current services negotiations, which began in 2000, are expected to widen the sector coverage of current schedules and deepen the level of existing commitments. The negotiations present a potential for expanded trade in health services as well as an opportunity to attract foreign direct investment and make it responsive to national health priorities. In many developing countries, this offers opportunities to acquire health services unavailable domestically, or to export health services and human resources to a larger world market. However, a number of concerns have been raised.

31. Some public health advocates fear, for instance, that the negotiations will force governments to open up their publicly funded health services to private, for-profit foreign investors. However, there is no obligation on any WTO Member to allow foreign supply of any particular service, nor even to guarantee domestic competition. Nor have the current services negotiations any particular implication for services provided in the exercise of governmental authority, which are exempted from the GATS. Also, developing countries are guaranteed "appropriate flexibility ... for opening fewer sectors, liberalizing fewer types of transactions, and progressively extending market access in line with their development situation".

Food security and nutrition

32. The issue of food security is complex and has many components. At the national level, economic access to food is critically dependent on national production and distribution, access to international markets and the availability of foreign exchange to buy imports. National food security is a concern primarily in countries that rely on imports of basic foods. In such countries, trade liberalization may reduce *self-sufficiency* in basic food production, and increases reliance on imports. However, this is not the same as worsening national *food security*, which is affected primarily by a country's ability to earn enough foreign exchange to import the food it needs.

33. The ongoing WTO negotiations on agriculture represent an opportunity to advance the agricultural trade and food security agenda, and developing countries have participated actively in these negotiations. Food security and related issues are being addressed in several ways in these negotiations. For example, a wide range of countries have called for the elimination of export subsidies and other forms of agricultural subsidization so as to put an end to their adverse impact on the production systems of developing countries. In addition, a group of developing countries has emphasized the need

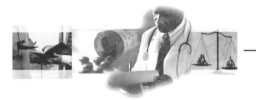

to give developing countries additional flexibilities to address their food security concerns, including flexibility to support their own production of essential food crops and for such assistance to be exempt from any reduction commitment. In general, increased market access is important for many, especially lower-income developing countries for which export agriculture remains the principal source of foreign exchange.

Emerging issues

34. There are two important technological advances that have the potential to revolutionize health care - biotechnology and information technology. A third emerging health issue is related, paradoxically, to the centuries-old use of herbal medicines and traditional knowledge for treating illnesses. The report examines the relationship between health and trade in these three cases.

35. Though the term covers a wide range of activities, *biotechnology* can be generally defined as "the application of scientific and engineering principles to the processing of materials by biological agents to provide goods and services" (OCDE, 1982). Biotechnology has already made enormous contributions to biomedical research and is beginning to translate into real-world applications in disease prevention and treatment. But as the scope of its application grows wider, from human and animals to genes and viruses to plants and trees, its impact on society and on economies is also widening. Biotechnology-related issues have been discussed in the WTO context. For example, the TRIPS Council has debated whether some biotechnological innovations are patentable, i.e. whether they meet the basic criteria of novelty, inventiveness and usefulness. There have also been some discussions in the TBT Committee regarding the GMO labelling requirements of various countries. And issues relating to food safety and to the potential spread of genetically modified seeds into the environment have been addressed by the SPS Committee in its discussions with respect to the Cartagena Biosafety Protocol. The SPS Committee has also discussed concerns raised with regard to some WTO Members' SPS notifications dealing with proposed GMO-related sanitary measures, as well as measures introduced without notification to the WTO.

36. *Information technology* is transforming societies and many economies, raising job productivity, creating new jobs, and speeding up communication and information flows, and the potential is still enormous. It has already stimulated changes in health care delivery, and has the potential to foster greater cross-border supply of health services.

In the longer term, information technology allowing real-time three-dimensional control of precision instruments with operator feedback may even support the remote perform-ance of surgical procedures. Its use in cross-border trade to serve the poor, however, could be constrained by high cost and lack of infrastructure and trained personnel.

37. As for *traditional medicine*, the knowledge of medicinal plants and their healing properties has been built up over centuries. Large segments of the population in the developing world continue to rely on them, while demand is growing among people in industrialized nations, contributing to growing international trade in herbal medicines. As the economic and trade value of the knowledge of traditional medicine and medici-nal plants increases, there is increasing concern about protecting it adequately and ensuring that the ensuing benefits are fairly and equitably shared.

Towards health and trade policy coherence

38. The last chapter of the report deals with the need for greater interaction between trade and health policy makers and practitioners and greater mutual awareness of trade and health policies. As this report has shown, the rules and provisions of the WTO Agreements most relevant to health generally permit countries to manage trade in goods and services in order to achieve their national health objectives, as long as health measures respect basic trade principles such as non-discrimination. Even these provi-sions may be waived under exceptions for public health. Yet concerns have been expressed by some observers that WTO rules could constitute a threat to sound public health policies.

39. A constructive way to address such concerns is to view them as opportunities for finding common ground. Minimizing possible conflicts between trade and health, and maximizing their mutual benefits, is an example of policy coherence. Thus, the chapter addresses the issue of coherence between health and trade policies at the national and international level. It describes efforts in two countries - Canada and Thailand - direct-ed towards health-and-trade policy coherence at the national level. And it examines efforts to coordinate activities at the international level between WHO and the WTO.

40. As the report went to print, the importance of the trade and health interlinkages and the need for greater coherence between trade and health policies received a strong endorsement from the international community at the Doha Ministerial Conference. The

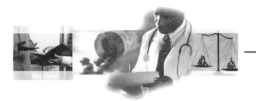

Doha Declaration on the TRIPS Agreements and Public Health and paragraph 6 of the Doha Ministerial Declaration made clear that WTO rules and health policies can go hand in hand, that public health considerations are important in implementing WTO rules, and that trade and health policies can be made mutually supportive. It was the intention of WHO and the WTO Secretariat in preparing this joint report to illustrate, for some key trade and health issues, that such coherence can be attained.

I. INTRODUCTION

1. Trade, the exchange of goods, services and information between individuals or groups, is as old as human history. Expanding trade is a central component of the increasing connectedness among countries.

2. Trade liberalization can affect health in multiple ways. Sometimes the impact is direct and the effect is obvious, as when a disease crosses a border together with a traded good. Other times the effects of trade liberalization are more indirect. For example, reducing tariffs may lead to lower prices for medical equipment and health-related products; changing international rules concerning patent protection may affect the prices of medicines and vaccines; importantly also, there is a positive link between freer trade and economic growth, which can lead to reduced poverty and higher standards of living, including better health.

3. The WHO defines health as "a state of complete physical, mental and social well-being and not merely the absence of disease or infirmity". "Public health" refers to all organized measures (whether public or private) to prevent disease, promote health, and prolong life of the population as a whole. Good health for all populations is an accepted international development goal and one building block for sustainable economic development, which is a goal both the World Health Organization and the World Trade Organization are working towards.

4. At the national level, health policy makers are increasingly interested in the two-way connection between trade and health. The principal objective of this report is to describe the actual and potential linkages between relevant WTO agreements and health so as to enable both trade and health officials to better understand, and monitor the effect of, these linkages. It does this by focusing on eight health issues:
(a) infectious disease control;
(b) food safety;
(c) tobacco;
(d) environment;
(e) access to drugs;
(f) health services;
(g) food security and nutrition; and,
(h) emerging issues (such as biotechnology).

5. The eight specific "health issues" listed above do not have separate WTO agreements that apply to them (with the exception of food safety). This report attempts to address only those WTO rules and agreements that are *most* relevant to each of these health issues. It illustrates key areas where trade rules may either complement or conflict with national public health policies. The conclusion emphasizes the need for policy coherence between health and trade at the national and international level and identifies opportunities to achieve greater coherence in health and trade policies in support of health and development goals.

6. The report is for readers with limited knowledge of health-and-trade issues. It does not delve deeply into fine details of the debate; the objective is to explain the issues and the various views in a factual manner. Those who wish to understand the nuances of WTO agreements and case law, keep up-to-date on current health-and-trade debates, or pursue particular topics in greater detail can contact the organizations directly and access the resources in the Annex.

7. The report contains three main Chapters. After this introduction, Chapter II examines WTO rules relevant to health, Chapter III analyzes the relationship between trade rules and some specific health issues and Chapter IV discusses proposals for enhancing policy coherence. The reader interested in a specific health issue may also begin by reading the relevant section in Chapter III and then go to Chapter II for more details on specific WTO Agreements.

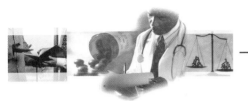

II. THE WTO AGREEMENTS RELEVANT TO HEALTH

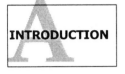

A. INTRODUCTION

(i) The institution

8. The World Trade Organization (WTO) is a relatively new international organization. However, it is responsible for a system that is over 50 years old. Established on 1 January 1995, the WTO replaced the General Agreement on Tariffs and Trade (GATT), which dated back to 1948. This was a consequence of a decision taken by governments after seven and a half years of negotiations (the "Uruguay Round"), which ended in 1994. With the WTO's creation, the rules were expanded to new areas. While the GATT dealt with trade in goods only, the WTO covers trade in services and intellectual property as well. There are also some areas, such as textiles, agriculture and sanitary and phytosanitary measures, where the WTO goes beyond the GATT by having established specific trade rules. Under the WTO, the procedure for settling trade disputes has also been strengthened.

9. The WTO is not a big institution. Like the WHO, it is based in Geneva but unlike the WHO it has no regional offices. It has a total staff of about 560 headed by a Director-General, and a limited budget.[1]

(ii) Structure

10. The WTO's top decision-making body is the Ministerial Conference which meets at least once every two years (see Chart 1). The General Council, which is normally attended by ambassadors and other Geneva-based delegates, or capital-based officials (who may include health experts), meets several times a year in the Geneva headquarters. The General Council also meets as the Trade Policy Review Body and the Dispute Settlement Body (DSB). Delegates at the day-to-day meetings of the WTO are government representatives of all WTO Members and representatives of observer organizations. Both during negotiations and in the WTO committee work, decisions are made by consensus. Voting is possible but it has never been used in the WTO.

---

[1]. The budget of the WTO is 143 million Swiss francs. The WHO has an annual budget of about US$1.1 billion and a Secretariat staff of 3,800, working in headquarters (Geneva), six regional offices, and some 150 countries (country offices/operations).

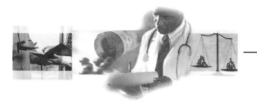

(iii) Objective

11. The objective of the WTO is illustrated by the preamble to the Agreement Establishing the World Trade Organization (the WTO Agreement), signed in Marrakesh in April 1994:

"Recognizing that their relations in the field of trade and economic endeavour should be conducted with a view to <u>raising standards of living</u>, ensuring full employment and a large and steadily growing volume of real income and effective demand, and expanding the production of and trade in goods and services, while allowing for the optimal use of the world's resources in accordance with the objective of <u>sustainable development</u>, seeking both to protect and preserve the environment and to enhance the means for doing so in a manner consistent with their respective needs and concerns at different levels of economic development, ..." [emphasis added]

(iv) Basic function

12. One of the key functions of the WTO is to serve as a forum for trade negotiations. The last round of multilateral trade negotiations was the Uruguay Round (1986-94). The WTO facilitates the implementation, administration and operation of the various covered agreements; however, the power of initiative in the context of the Organization rests not with the Secretariat but with Member governments whose representatives constitute and preside over the many councils and committees dealing with issues that arise in connection with the agreements.

13. The WTO is not a funding organization; it has no mandate to finance development projects. Nevertheless, the WTO does provide technical assistance to developing countries. The aim of this assistance is both to assist Members in the implementation of WTO agreements and to train officials so that they understand the system and its agreements, know how to administer them, and negotiate more effectively. Technical assistance is also extended to acceding countries. The training is often rather "legal" and is aimed at providing an understanding of rights and obligations Members have under the various agreements

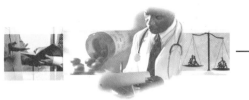

Chart 1: WTO Structure

All WTO Members may participate in all councils, committees, etc, except Appellate Body, Dispute Settlement panels, Textiles Monitoring Body, and plurilateral committees.

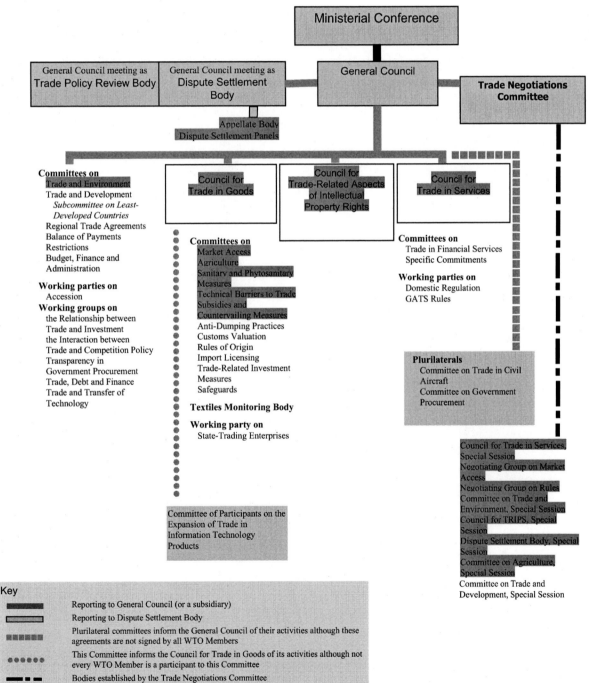

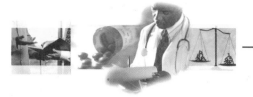

(v) Membership and accession

14. By February 2002, 144 countries were Members of the WTO. Together they account for more than 90 per cent of world trade. In the WTO, gaining membership is not automatic. Countries negotiate their accession to the WTO with existing Members. WTO agreements are, in general, ratified in Members' parliaments.

15. Currently, several countries are actively negotiating their entry into the organisation, including the Russian Federation. There is growing consensus that WTO membership constitutes a key step towards integrating developing countries into the global economy and the international trading system. Since WTO's establishment in 1995, over 40 developing countries have sought admission to the WTO. Many of these countries cite the benefits of the WTO accession process itself, which serves as an impetus to spur and consolidate their own internal reform process and accelerate their economic development (see, for instance, WTO document WT/MIN(01)/2 of 22 October 2001, p. 59 and p. 62).

16. Countries that wish to join the WTO must negotiate with existing WTO Members and a working party is set up to handle each application. Accession working parties are open to all WTO Members, and countries with an interest in the applicant country's trade join the working party. Acceding country governments must then undergo a fact-finding process regarding their trade policy and undertake a series of commitments to bring trade policy into line with the WTO agreements. The accession process can be quite burdensome, complicated, and lengthy. As of February 2002, 16 of the 44 governments that had applied for WTO membership had completed the process and become WTO Members. The entire process, which in some cases began before 1995 under the GATT, took between 3 and 10 years, except in the case of China, which recently became a Member after 15 years of accession negotiations.

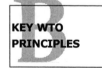

KEY WTO PRINCIPLES

B. KEY WTO PRINCIPLES

17. The rules for goods and services under the WTO share some common features. First, the broad principles are set out in the GATT (for goods), and the General Agreement on Trade in Services (GATS). In addition to this, there are specific agreements or, under GATS, annexes dealing with the special requirements of specific sectors or issues. For example, for trade in goods there are specific agreements relating to

quality and safety regulations. The GATS has several Annexes elaborating on the Agreement's coverage of, and application to, issues such as movements of natural persons and specific features of financial services (e.g. prudential standards) and telecommunications (e.g. access to and use of public networks and services). Both the GATT and the GATS are complemented by detailed and lengthy schedules (or lists) of commitments made by individual countries. In the goods area, these relate to tariff levels and, for agricultural products, also to subsidies. In services, the commitments specify the degree of foreign access which is guaranteed to foreign services and service providers in specific sectors, together with any limitations on market access and national treatment. It should be stressed that these are minimum conditions; nothing prevents a government from according better treatment than that guaranteed in its schedule. While treated differently in the GATT and the GATS, as well as in the specific agreements and Annexes, the key principles of most-favoured-nation (MFN) and national treatment are a common feature.

(i) Most-favoured-nation (MFN): treating other WTO Members equally

18. Under the WTO agreements, countries cannot normally discriminate between their trading partners. In simple terms, a special benefit granted to one country (such as a lower customs tariffs for one of their products) has to be granted to all other WTO Members. This principle, known as most-favoured-nation (MFN) treatment, is enshrined in Article I of the GATT, which governs trade in goods. MFN treatment is also one of core obligations of the GATS (Article II) and the Agreement on Trade-Related Aspects of Intellectual Property Rights (TRIPS) (Article 4). Together, those three Agreements cover the main areas of trade covered by the WTO. In general, MFN means that every time a country lowers (or introduces) a trade barrier or opens up a market, it has to do so for the same goods or services or service suppliers from all its fellow WTO Members - whether rich or poor, weak or strong.

(ii) National treatment: treating foreigners and locals equally

19. The principle of national treatment requires that imported and locally-produced goods be treated equally, in terms of competitive opportunities in the importing country's market. The same applies to foreign and domestic services and service suppliers, and to foreign and local nationals in regard to the protection of intellectual property. This principle is found in all the three main WTO Agreements (Article 3 of GATT,

Article XVII of GATS and Article 3 of TRIPS), although the principle is handled differently in each of these Agreements. National treatment under GATT only applies once a product has entered the market. Therefore, charging customs duty on an import is not a violation of national treatment even if locally-produced products are not charged an equivalent duty. Under the GATS, national treatment is not a general obligation. It applies only to sectors listed in the individual Members' schedule of commitments. Moreover, Members may specify in their schedules any differential treatment they wish to apply to foreign services and service suppliers as compared to nationals. An unqualified commitment means that they will be treated in the same way as nationals. Under TRIPS, the principle requires foreign nationals to be given no less favourable treatment than that given to a country's own nationals in regard to the protection of intellectual property.

(iii) The MFN principle and public health

20. How is the MFN principle applied in practice? For example, health authorities in a country may decide to restrict the level of pesticides on fruit because of an unacceptable health risk. This will affect trade to the extent that imported fruit does not meet the specified requirement. This is a perfectly legitimate health concern translated into a regulatory action at the border, which, if applied in a non-discriminatory way, and based on scientific principles, is a justifiable trade barrier under WTO rules. In respect of discrimination, if the intention is to protect the consumer, it should not matter where the health risk originates, unless there is evidence that some countries have a higher level of risk. The point is that the requirement has to be the same, irrespective of where the product originates. Fruit from countries that do not fulfil the sanitary requirement could, justifiably, be banned. But the same fruit with an acceptable level of pesticide residues would be allowed in.

(iv) Health exceptions in GATT and GATS

21. Since the inception of GATT more than 50 years ago, Article XX of GATT guarantees the Members' right to take measures to restrict imports and exports of products when those measures are necessary to protect the health of humans, animals and plants (Article XX(b)) or otherwise relate to the conservation of natural resources (Article XX(g)). In a similar vein, Article XIV of the GATS authorizes Members to take measures to restrict services and service suppliers for the protection of human, animal or plant life or health. If the relevant conditions are met, including the good faith obli-

gations inherent in the chapeaux of these Articles, they provide an override of any other obligations, including tariff concessions on goods or specific commitments on services, that WTO Members have undertaken under WTO Agreements. These provisions recognize that there are cases where Members may wish to pursue other legitimate policy objectives, such as health. The health exceptions allowed for in GATT and GATS indicate the importance that WTO Members assign to national autonomy in the protection of health. TRIPS does not contain an exception for health purposes per se, but it does allow measures necessary to protect public health and nutrition, provided they are consistent with other TRIPS provisions (TRIPS, Article 8 - Principles).[2]

22. The WTO jurisprudence has clearly established that WTO Members have the right to determine the level of health protection they deem appropriate; the same principle has been reiterated in the Agreement on Technical Barriers to Trade (TBT Agreement) and the Agreement on the Application of Sanitary and Phytosanitary Measures (SPS Agreement) for the specific measures covered by those Agreements. It is also clear that there is no requirement under Article XX of the GATT 1994 to quantify, as such, the risk to human life or health. As with the SPS Agreement, risk under Article XX of the GATT 1994 may be evaluated either in quantitative or qualitative terms.

23. To make use of the health exceptions, WTO Agreements generally require the health measures be no more trade-restrictive than necessary. Determining whether a measure is "necessary" involves a process of weighing and balancing a series of factors which include the importance of the interests protected by the measure, its efficacy in pursuing the policies, and its impact on imports or exports. The more vital or important the policies, the easier it would be to accept as "necessary" a measure designed for that purpose. Human health has been recognized by the WTO as being "important in the highest degree."[3]

24. Stepping away from the general principles of non-discrimination and exceptions, the following three sub-sections look at how more specific trade rules apply these principles to the areas of technical barriers to trade, intellectual property and services as they relate to health.

---

[2] See also the Ministerial Declaration on the TRIPS Agreement and Public Health, WTO document WT/MIN(01)/DEC/2, which is reproduced below in section 3.

[3] European Communities - Measures Affecting Asbestos and Asbestos-containing Products, Report of the Appellate Body, WT/DS135/AB/R, 12 March 2001, Para. 172.

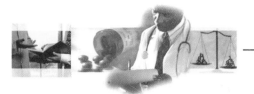

TECHNICAL BARRIERS TO TRADE

C. TECHNICAL BARRIERS TO TRADE

25. WTO rules which govern technical barriers to trade applied for reasons of protecting human health are covered by either the Agreement on Technical Barriers to Trade (TBT Agreement) or the Agreement on the Application of Sanitary and Phytosanitary Measures (SPS Agreement). Under both these agreements, health is considered a legitimate objective for restricting trade.

1. The TBT Agreement

26. Technical barriers to trade were first addressed in the Tokyo Round of multilateral trade negotiations (1973-1979). The "old" TBT Agreement, referred to as the "Standards Code", came into force in 1980. This was a plurilateral agreement to which only 46 countries adhered. The new TBT Agreement, which came into force with the WTO in 1995, is binding on all WTO Members. It contains more stringent obligations than the preceding version of the agreement.

(i) Overall objective, purpose of Agreement, and scope

27. All Members have the right to restrict trade for "legitimate objectives" under the TBT Agreement. These legitimate objectives include the protection of human health or safety, the protection of animal or plant life or health, the protection of the environment, national security interests, and the prevention of deceptive practices. The TBT Agreement aims to ensure that product requirements, and procedures that are used to assess compliance with those requirements, do not create unnecessary obstacles to trade. In other words, the TBT Agreement allows countries to obstruct trade for legitimate reasons, including health, but its principles require that such measures do not unnecessarily restrict trade. The Agreement applies to product requirements that are mandatory ("technical regulations") as well as voluntary ("standards"). It covers such requirements developed by governments or private entities, whether at the national or the regional level.[4]

[4.] Annex 1, paragraphs 1 and 2 of the TBT Agreement defines these two concepts.

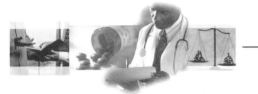

(ii) Principles

28. The Agreement lays out a number of principles. The first is non-discrimination. With respect to technical requirements, non-discrimination means that if a Member applies certain requirements to imported products, it has to apply the same requirements to like domestic products (national treatment). If it applies a requirement to imports from one source, it has to apply it to like imports from all other sources as well (most-favoured-nation treatment).

29. Members should also seek to avoid unnecessary obstacles to trade. In practice, this means that Members must design technical requirements in the way that is not more trade restrictive than necessary to fulfill a legitimate objective, making them proportional to the objectives which they are trying to fulfil. Members are also encouraged to base their measures on international standards. The use of international standards helps to avoid the creation of multiple types of technical requirements and conformity assessment procedures at the national level, which can obstruct trade.

(iii) Examples as applied to health

30. Protection of human, animal, plant and environmental health are among the legitimate objectives for which product requirements may be developed. Of all TBT regulations notified to the WTO in 2000, the largest single group (254 notifications, out of the total of 725 that were received) had human health or safety as their objective. For example, one Member notified regulations related to radio communications equipment which reduce human exposure to electromagnetic radiation. Another Member notified a regulation which limited the substances that are used in cosmetics and may cause allergies. Still another Member notified a measure that regulated the use of chemicals that may cause occupational health hazards. Measures taken for the protection of animal and plant life or health usually fall under the SPS Agreement, and therefore only 10 TBT notifications had these objectives.

(iv) Use of international health standards

31. While the TBT Agreement strongly encourages the use of international standards, Members may depart from them if they consider that their application would be ineffective or inappropriate for the fulfilment of certain legitimate objectives. If a Member considers certain WHO standards appropriate to be adopted as national standards or

technical regulations, it should use them. Nevertheless, Members are free to set standards at a level they consider appropriate, but have to be able to justify their decisions if requested by another Member to do so. The Agreement also calls upon Members to play an active role in the process of international standardisation, particularly for any product for which it is developing a national requirement.

(v) Review of the TBT Agreement

32. Article 15.4 of the TBT Agreement states that "Not later than the end of the third year from the date of entry into force of the WTO Agreement and at the end of each of three-year period thereafter, the Committee shall review the operation and implementation of this Agreement." The Agreement has been reviewed under this provision twice, and the Second Triennial Review was concluded on 13 November 2000. The review examined the operation of the Agreement with respect to notifications, obligations and procedures for information exchange, the use of international standards, guides and recommendations, conformity assessment procedures the provision of technical assistance, and more.

33. One of the most relevant outcomes of the review was the adoption of a "Decision of the Committee on Principles for the Development of International Standards, Guides and Recommendations." The Decision calls upon international standardizing bodies to observe a certain number of principles in their work, which include: transparency, openness, impartiality and consensus, effectiveness and relevance, and coherence. It also calls upon them to take the development dimension into account in the elaboration of their standards, guides and recommendations. International standardizing bodies that fulfil these criteria will be considered "international" within the meaning of the TBT Agreement. [5]

2. The SPS Agreement

(i) Rationale for the SPS Agreement

34. The SPS Agreement is linked to the Uruguay Round negotiations on the Agreement on Agriculture. In seeking to reduce agricultural tariffs and subsidies, some Members were concerned that countries might turn to the use of non-tariff barriers to protect domestic agricultural sectors; it could be tempting to use human, animal or plant

---

[5.] The Decision can be consulted in document G/TBT/9 available of the WTO website.

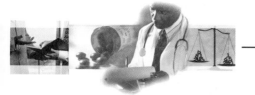

health as an excuse to restrict trade. Such measures could negate many of the benefits from reducing tariffs and subsidies. This led to the negotiation of the Agreement on the application of such types of measures, known as sanitary and phytosanitary measures (or "SPS measures"). [6]

(ii) SPS directly relevant to health

35. The SPS Agreement contains specific rules for countries which want to restrict trade to ensure food safety and the protection of human life from plant- or animal-carried diseases (zoonoses). Its objective is two-fold. It aims to (i) recognize the sovereign right of Members to determine the level of health protection they deem appropriate; and (ii) ensure that a sanitary or phytosanitary requirement does not represent an unnecessary, arbitrary, scientifically unjustifiable, or disguised restriction on international trade. In order to achieve its objective, the SPS Agreement encourages Members to use international standards, guidelines and recommendations where they exist. Members may adopt SPS measures which result in higher levels of health protection - or measures aimed at health concerns for which international standards do not exist - provided that they are scientifically justified.

(iii) Difference in coverage compared to TBT Agreement

36. To assess whether the SPS or TBT Agreement is relevant to any given technical barrier to trade, the fundamental question to be posed is: what is the purpose of the measure. In other words, whether a any given measure is an SPS measure will depend on whether its objective fits in any of the four categories set out in Box 1 below.

---

[6] This is not to say that there were no rules relevant to sanitary and phytosanitary measures prior to the WTO SPS Agreement. The 1979 TBT greement applied to those countries which were members of it. The GATT 1947 also applied. As discussed above, the GATT Article XX(b) xemption for measures necessary to protect human, animal or plant life or health is directly relevant. However, the SPS Agreement lends 1ore precision to this area, in which, prior to 1995, the rules were fairly general.

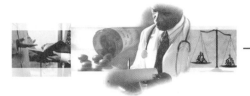

Box 1
The definition of an SPS measure at a glance

Measures taken to protect:	from:
human or animal life	additives, contaminants, toxins or disease-causing organisms in their food, beverages, feedstuffs;
human life	plant- or animal-carried diseases (zoonoses);
animal or plant life	pests, diseases, or disease-causing organisms
a country	damage caused by the entry, establishment or spread of pests (including invasive species).

---

37. If the measure does not fit the definition in the above box, it is likely to be a TBT measure. While there is no overlap in coverage between the two Agreements, sometimes the same government regulation contains both SPS and TBT measures.[7] Examples of SPS measures include the following: (i) requiring animals and animal products to come from disease-free areas; (ii) inspection of products for microbiological contaminants; (iii) mandating a specific fumigation treatment for products; and (iv) setting maximum allowable levels of pesticide residues in food.

(iv) Why is it important which Agreement applies?

38. While the aim of preventing unnecessary trade barriers is common to both the SPS and TBT Agreements, the rights and obligations they entail are quite different. Under the SPS Agreement, measures may be imposed only to the extent necessary to protect life or health, on the basis of scientific information. However, the TBT Agreement permits the introduction of technical regulations to meet a variety of legitimate objectives, including national security, the prevention of deceptive practices, protection of human health or safety or the environment. Essentially, the WTO recognizes that governments will impose technical requirements for a wide variety of reasons, and the TBT Agreement allows them to do this, subject to certain disciplines.

---

[7] The distinction here is purely legal. In practice, technical regulations being developed by governments do not always treat safety and quality issues separately. For example, a regulation on labelling might address both safety issues and information about content. Such a requirement would have to be notified under both Agreements; the "safety" element would fall under the SPS Agreement and the "content" element would fall under the TBT Agreement.

39. The SPS Agreement applies to a narrowly defined range of health protection measures, but places quite strict requirements on these measures: for example, they have to be based on a scientific justification. The TBT Agreement, on the other hand, applies to a wide range of technical requirements, and solely notes that available scientific information may be one of the relevant elements of consideration in assessing risks. Some of these technical requirements are introduced for health or safety purposes, but others are introduced to standardize products, ensure quality or avoid consumer deception. In these cases scientific information might be less relevant in assessing risks than, for example, processing technology and intended end-uses.

40. If a trade dispute arises, the question of which of the two agreements applies can make a difference. While several disputes on SPS measures have arisen, and three have gone through the full panel process, there is no jurisprudence on the TBT Agreement yet.

(v) Scientific justification

41. A fundamental requirement of the SPS Agreement is that Members have to be able to demonstrate, on the basis of scientific evidence, that there is indeed a risk to health which justifies trade measures not based on international standards. Members have a basic obligation to ensure that SPS measures are applied only to the extent necessary to protect human, animal or plant life or health and are not maintained without sufficient scientific evidence except in certain circumstances, as described in the next paragraph. The SPS Agreement encourages the use of international standards. In the area of food safety, the SPS Agreement explicitly recognizes the international standards developed by the joint FAO/WHO Codex Alimentarius Commission. This means that if a government has based its requirement, such as a maximum residue level for a pesticide in a food, on a Codex standard, it is presumed to be meeting its WTO obligations.[8]

(vi) Provisional measures

42. Available scientific evidence is not always sufficient for an objective assessment of risk to human, animal or plant life or health. In such circumstances, the SPS Agreement permits the adoption of provisional measures on the basis of the available pertinent information about the health risk of a product or process. However, when taking such a provisional measure, a Member must seek the additional information necessary for a

The main articles in the SPS Agreement relevant to scientific justification are Articles 2 and 5.

more objective risk assessment, and review the SPS measure within a reasonable period of time. Provisional measures could be taken, for example, as an emergency response to a sudden outbreak of an animal disease suspected of being linked to imports.

(vii) Review

43. The SPS Agreement was reviewed in 1998. At the Doha Ministerial Conference in November 2001, Ministers instructed the SPS Committee to review the operation of the Agreement at least once every four years. Any further review will be undertaken "as the need arises" (Article 12.7).[9] WTO Members working through the SPS Committee may submit proposals to amend the text of this Agreement in light of further experience gained in its implementation, although this has not happened to date. "Food safety" is one issue on the table in the context of the on-going negotiations under the Agreement on Agriculture. It is too early in the negotiations to say how, if at all, this may affect the SPS Agreement.

D. INTELLECTUAL PROPERTY AND TRADE (TRIPS)

44. The TRIPS Agreement requires WTO Members to establish minimum standards for protecting and enforcing intellectual property rights. Its objectives are set out in Article 7:

The protection and enforcement of intellectual property rights should contribute to the promotion of technological innovation and to the transfer and dissemination of technology, to the mutual advantage of producers and users of technological knowledge and in a manner conducive to social and economic welfare, and to a balance of rights and obligations.

45. The principles of the TRIPS Agreement are set out in its Article 8:

1. Members may, in formulating or amending their laws and regulations, adopt measures necessary to protect public health and nutrition, and to promote the public interest in sectors of vital importance to their socio-economic and technological development, provided that such measures are consistent with the provisions of this Agreement.

---

[9] The revision of the SPS Agreement is contained in document G/SPS/12, available at www.wto.org. The matter of further reviews is currently one of the issues under consideration in the Implementation Review Mechanism under the auspices of the General Council.

2. Appropriate measures, provided that they are consistent with the provisions of this Agreement, may be needed to prevent the abuse of intellectual property rights by right holders or the resort to practices which unreasonably restrain trade or adversely affect the international transfer of technology.

46. Thus, the TRIPS Agreement attempts to strike a balance between the longer term objective of providing incentives for future inventions and creations, and the shorter term objective of allowing people to use existing inventions and creations. The Agreement covers a wide range of subjects, from copyright, patents and trademarks to integrated circuit designs and trade secrets.[10]

47. The TRIPS Agreement provides some flexibility for governments to fine-tune the basic balance provided for in the Agreement in the light of national social, developmental and other public policy objectives (see section III). While its rules require that national legislation embody certain minimum standards of protection, they afford considerable discretion in how these are implemented in practice. In each area of intellectual property, it allows governments to provide for exceptions, exclusions and limitations to rights, such as in the case of national emergencies, public non-commercial use, or remedying anti-competitive practices. This can be done, for example, in the form of compulsory licensing, exhaustion regimes and other types of exceptions, provided certain conditions are fulfilled.

What is relevant to health in the TRIPS Agreement?

48. The areas of intellectual property covered by the TRIPS Agreement that are relevant to health include: patents; trademarks including service marks, which are relevant, for example, to combating counterfeit drugs; and undisclosed information, including trade secrets and test data (see box 2). In respect of each of these areas, the Agreement sets out the minimum standards of protection that must be adopted by each Member. Each of the main elements of protection is defined, namely the subject matter to be protected, the rights to be conferred and permissible exceptions to those rights, and the minimum duration of protection. The standards build on those in the main pre-existing WIPO Conventions, substantive provisions of which are incorporated into the Agreement by reference. While the focus here is on patents, this is only one part of the TRIPS Agreement. One of the purposes of the TRIPS Agreement is, for

10. Intellectual property protection is also covered by international treaties developed under the auspices of the World Intellectual Property Organization (WIPO). WIPO administers 11 treaties that set out internationally agreed rights and common standards for IPR protection, that the States which sign them agree to apply within their own territories. See WIPO's website, listed in the Annex, for further information.

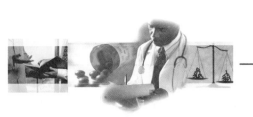

instance, also to provide for more effective international cooperation against counterfeiting, including international trade in counterfeit goods, such as drugs (see box 3).

Box 2
The relevance of trademarks and "undisclosed information" to health

• **Trademarks**. The agreement defines what types of signs must be eligible for protection as trademarks, and what the minimum rights conferred on their owners must be. It says that service marks must be protected in the same way as trademarks used for goods. Marks that have become well-known in a particular country enjoy additional protection.

• **"Undisclosed information"**. Trade secrets and other types of "undisclosed information" which have commercial value must be protected against breach of confidence and other acts contrary to honest commercial practices. But reasonable steps must be taken to keep the information secret. In the area of pharmaceuticals, certain production processes could be protected under trade secrets. Test data submitted to governments in order to obtain marketing approval for new pharmaceuticals (or agricultural chemicals) must also be protected against unfair commercial use.

Box 3
Counterfeit drugs

There have been cases of counterfeiting of both patented and non-patended drugs. Counterfeit drugs, which often contain few or no active ingredients and may actually be harmful to health, are a major problem in many developing countries, notably in sub-Saharan Africa. Counterfeit drugs are recognized as a problem undermining the effectiveness of drug therapy. Many of the counterfeit products on local markets in these countries are imported rather than locally produced. The TRIPS Agreement addresses this issue in three main ways.

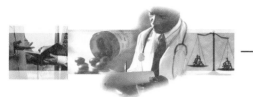

Box 3
Counterfeit drugs (cont'd)

• First, it ensures that owners of trademarks are able to obtain protection for their trademarks under the law of each WTO Member.

• Second, it specifies the procedures and remedies that must be available so that right holders can secure effective enforcement of their rights against infringing activity. Civil judicial procedures and remedies must be available against any infringing activity, but some additional avenues of recourse have to be available against counterfeiting. These are actions which involve the assistance of the customs administration to prevent imports of counterfeit products and criminal penalties where counterfeiting is taking place wilfully and on a commercial scale.

• Third, to support effective national solutions to this problem, the TRIPS Agreement provides for international cooperation to fight counterfeiting by promoting the exchange of information and cooperation between customs authorities with regard to trade in counterfeit trademark goods (See Article 69 of the TRIPS Agreement entitled "International Cooperation).

(i) Provisions for public health protection

49. Patent protection for pharmaceutical products is an area where the problem of finding a proper balance is particularly acute - namely, between the goal of providing incentives for future inventions of new drugs and the goal of affordable access to existing drugs. It is especially important from a social and public health point of view that new drugs and vaccines to treat and prevent diseases are generated, and that the incentives provided by the patent system effectively promote this. Precisely because of the social value of the drugs so generated, they need to be widely accessible as quickly as possible.

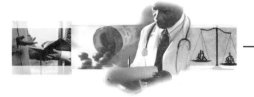

50. The patent system provides for, on the one hand, exclusive rights granted to inventors of new drugs, and, on the other hand, the requirement that for a new drug to benefit from such rights (to be patentable), it must be new, involve an inventive step, be industrially applicable and be fully disclosed, and further that after a term of protection the invention will fall into the public domain and become free and useable by all.

51. In addition, the TRIPS Agreement contains several other provisions enabling governments to implement their intellectual property regimes in a manner which takes account of immediate and longer-term public health considerations. Article 8 explicitly recognizes the right of WTO Members to "adopt measures necessary to protect public health and nutrition, and to promote the public interest in sectors of vital importance to their socio-economic and technological development, provided that such measures are consistent with the provisions of this Agreement." Furthermore, the TRIPS Agreement provides for certain exemptions from patentability, the possibility to make limited exceptions to patent owners' exclusive rights, compulsory licensing, and parallel importation. These are discussed in greater detail below.

(ii) What are Member governments' obligations with respect to pharmaceutical patents under TRIPS?

52. International conventions before TRIPS did not usually specify the minimum standards for patents. Over 40 countries provided no product patent protection for pharmaceuticals prior to the launching of the negotiation of the TRIPS Agreement and some 20 WTO Members still did not do so by the time of the conclusion of the TRIPS negotiations. A few of these countries did not provide process protection in this area as well. The duration of patents was less than 20 years in many countries. TRIPS rules require WTO Members to provide patent protection for any invention, whether a product (such as a medicine) or a process (such as a method of producing the chemical ingredients for a medicine), while allowing certain exceptions. Patent protection has to last at least 20 years from the date the patent application was filed.[11]

---

11. In the case of pharmaceutical products, which are subjected to lengthy procedures that verify safety and efficacy, the effective patent life remaining out of the 20 years once the product has received marketing approval is generally considerably shorter. For example, in the WTO dispute between the European Communities and Canada regarding Patent Protection of Pharmaceutical Products (WT/DS114/R, para. 7.3), it was accepted by the parties to this dispute that the effective patent life was typically in the region of 8 to 12 years. Most industrialized countries allow patent term extension for pharmaceuticals to compensate for such regulatory approval delays but this is not a requirement under TRIPS.

53. As in other WTO Agreements, non-discrimination is a core TRIPS principle. With some exceptions, Members must not discriminate on the basis of the nationality of persons or companies (Articles 3, 4 and 5). In addition, Members cannot discriminate between different fields of technology in the availability and enjoyment of patent rights. Nor can they discriminate in these areas on the basis of the place of invention and whether products are imported or locally produced (Article 27.1).

54. Three substantive criteria have to be met if an invention is to qualify for a patent:

(a)   it has to be new ("novelty");
(b)   it must involve an "inventive step" (it must not be obvious); and,
(c)   it must have "industrial applicability" (it must be useful).

55. Moreover, details of the invention have to be described in the application and therefore have to be made public. This is referred to as "disclosure". Disclosure has to be sufficient to enable a person skilled in the area to reproduce the invention. Members may also require the patent applicant to reveal the best method for carrying it out.

56. As the TRIPS Agreement does not define the terms "new", "inventive step" and "non-obvious", national patent laws vary in how they construe these terms for the purposes of evaluating patent applications. Patentability standards which are too lax can make it possible to obtain protection for relatively minor innovations. Some concern has been expressed that this can facilitate what is sometimes referred to as "evergreening" of pharmaceutical patents, meaning that improved versions of the original drug may stay under patent protection even after the original version has fallen into the public domain. Very strict criteria may make it more difficult for small and medium-sized enterprises to use the patent system, especially in developing countries.

57. Regarding eligibility for patenting, governments can refuse to grant patents for three reasons that may relate to public health:

(a) inventions whose commercial exploitation needs to be prevented to protect human, animal or plant life or health;

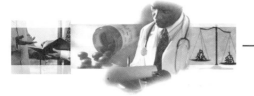

(b) diagnostic, therapeutic and surgical methods for treating humans or animals;

(c) plant and animal inventions other than micro-organisms, and essentially biological processes for the production of plants or animals other than non-biological and micro-biological processes.

(iii) A patent is not a permit to put a product on a market

58. Patents provide the patent owner with the legal means to prevent others from making, using, or selling the new invention for a limited period of time, subject to a number of exceptions. It is not, however, a permit to put a product on the market. A patent only gives an inventor the right to prevent others from using the patented invention. It says nothing about whether the product is safe or therapeutic for consumers and whether it can be supplied. Patented pharmaceuticals still have to go through rigorous testing and approval before they can be put on the market.

(iv) Research exception and "Bolar" provisions

59. Under the TRIPS Agreement, governments can make limited exceptions to patent rights provided certain conditions are met. These exceptions must not "unreasonably" conflict with the "normal" exploitation of the patent and must not unreasonably prejudice the legitimate interests of the patent owner, taking into account the legitimate interest of third parties (Article 30). A range of exceptions may be covered by this provision. For example, many countries provide for a "research" or "experimental use" exception to allow researchers to use a patented invention for research, in order to understand the invention more fully. In addition, Article 30 permits countries to allow manufacturers of generic drugs to use the patented invention, without the patent owner's permission and before the patent protection expires, for the purpose of obtaining marketing approval from public health authorities. Generic producers are thus able to market their versions almost as soon as the patent expires. This provision is sometimes called the "regulatory exception" or "Bolar" provision, and has been upheld as conforming with the TRIPS Agreement in a WTO dispute ruling: in a report adopted on 7 April 2000, a WTO dispute settlement panel stated that Canadian law was consistent with the TRIPS Agreement in allowing manufacturers to do so.[12]

---

12. Canada - Patent Protection of Pharmaceutical Products, WT/DS114/R, dated 17 March 2000.

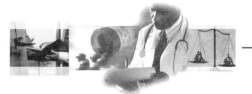

(v) Compulsory licensing and government use

60. Compulsory licensing takes place when a government allows a third party to produce a patented product or use a patented process without the consent of the patent owner. Most developed and developing countries provide for compulsory licensing in their national legislation. The term "compulsory licensing" does not appear in the TRIPS Agreement. Instead, the practice falls under "other use without authorization of the right holder" (Article 31), of which compulsory licensing is only part, since "other use" also includes use by governments for their own purposes. In current public discussion, compulsory licenses are usually associated with pharmaceuticals but could apply to patents in any field.

61. The TRIPS Agreement does not limit the reasons for which governments may grant compulsory licences. However, compulsory licensing or government use of a patent without the authorization of the right holder can only be done under a number of conditions aimed at protecting the legitimate interests of the patent holder. Article 31 lists a number of provisions that should be respected in such cases. For example, the person or company applying for a licence must have first attempted unsuccessfully to obtain a voluntary licence from the right holder on reasonable commercial terms. However, for "national emergencies", "other circumstances of extreme urgency", "public non-commercial use" or remedying anti-competitive practices, there is no need to try for a voluntary licence. If a compulsory licence is issued, adequate remuneration must still be paid to the patent holder, taking into account the economic value of the authorization (Article 31(h)). Compulsory licensing must meet several other requirements listed in the same Article. In particular, it cannot take the form of an exclusive licence, and "shall be authorized predominantly for the supply of the domestic market of the Member authorizing such use" (Article 31(f)). This condition need not be applied where such use is permitted to remedy a practice determined after judicial or administrative process to be anti-competitive (Article 31(k)).

(vi) Parallel imports and "exhaustion" of rights

62. Parallel importation is importation of a patented or trademarked product from a country where it is marketed either by the right holder or with his consent. In the TRIPS Agreement, this matter is regulated by the concept of the "exhaustion" of intellectual property rights. The TRIPS Agreement simply says (Article 6) that none of its provisions, except those dealing with non-discrimination on the basis of nationality

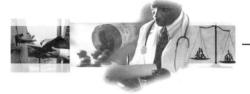

(national treatment and most-favoured-nation treatment), can be used to address the issue of exhaustion of intellectual property rights in a WTO dispute.

(vii) Developing countries' transition periods - Year 2000 for most

63. In general, developing countries and economies in transition from central planning did not have to implement most provisions of the TRIPS Agreement until 1 January 2000. Least-developed countries have at least until 1 January 2006, but this deadline may be extended. Developed countries had until 1 January 1996, one year after the TRIPS Agreement took effect, to apply it. Most new Members who joined after the WTO was created in 1995 have agreed to apply the TRIPS Agreement as soon as they joined. This question is determined by each new Member's terms of accession. The TRIPS Agreement specifically recognizes the economic, financial, administrative and technological constraints of the least-developed countries, and therefore provides the possibility for further extension of the transitional period. The recent Doha Declaration on the TRIPS Agreement and Public Health allows least-developed countries until 1 January 2016 to meet the TRIPS provisions on the protection of patents and undisclosed information with respect to pharmaceutical products, without prejudice to their right to seek other extensions of the transition periods (see below, section III, Box 18).

64. Some developing countries may delay patent protection for pharmaceutical products (and agricultural chemicals) until 1 January 2005, under provisions stating that a developing country that did not provide product patent protection in a particular area of technology when the TRIPS Agreement came into force (on 1 January 1995) has up to 10 years to introduce the protection. However, for pharmaceuticals and agricultural chemicals, countries eligible to use this provision (i.e. countries that did not provide such protection on 1 January 1995) have two obligations:

(a) They must allow inventors to file patent applications from 1 January 1995, even though the actual decision on whether or not to grant any patent need not be taken until the end of the transition period. (This is sometimes called the "mailbox" provision). This provision was established because the date of filing is significant, as it is used for assessing whether the application meets the criteria for patenting, including novelty ("newness" criterion).

(b) Second, if the government allows the relevant pharmaceutical or agricultural chemical product to be marketed during the transition period, it must - subject to certain conditions - provide the patent applicant an exclusive marketing right for the product for five years, or until a decision on a product patent is taken, whichever is shorter.

65. Fewer than 20 developing countries were affected by the provisions referred to in the previous paragraph, most having had product patent protection for pharmaceutical products all along or having introduced it prior to the entry into force of the TRIPS Agreement.[13]

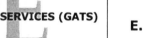

E. SERVICES (GATS)

66. In the past, most services were not considered to be tradable across borders. Much has occurred to alter the tradability of services, including health services. Advances in communications technology, including the development of e-commerce, as well as regulatory changes in many parts of the world have made it easier to deliver services across borders. In many countries, changes in government policy have left greater room for the private sector - domestic as well as foreign - to provide services. Partly as a result, services have become the fastest-growing segment of the world economy, providing more than 60 per cent of global output and employment.

67. Such changes led governments to include services in trade negotiations, resulting in the General Agreement on Trade in Services (GATS) at the end of the Uruguay Round. GATS takes a gradual approach to trade liberalization. So far, the liberalizing effects have remained limited as most WTO Members have made relatively few commitments that go beyond existing levels of access.

68. GATS recognizes the special nature of services compared to goods by defining four modes of service delivery. Box 4 describes each mode and gives health services examples.

13. To the best knowledge of the WTO Secretariat, these countries were Angola, Argentina, Bangladesh, Brazil, Cuba, Egypt, Guatemala, India, Kuwait, Madagascar, Morocco, Pakistan, Paraguay, Qatar, Tunisia, Turkey, United Arab Emirates and Uruguay. A number of these countries, including Argentina, Brazil, Guatemala, Morocco, Paraguay, Turkey and Uruguay, are not using the full transition period available to them, having already introduced product patent protection for pharmaceuticals or indicated their intention to do so prior to 1 January 2005.

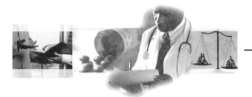

Box 4
Health applications of GATS services modes

Mode 1
Cross-border supply, e.g. provision of diagnosis or treatment planning services
in country A by suppliers in country B, via telecommunications ('telemedicine')

Mode 2
Consumption abroad, e.g. movement of patients from
country A to country B for treatment

Mode 3
Commercial presence, e.g. establishment of or investment in hospitals
in country A whose owners are from country B

Mode 4
Presence of natural persons, e.g. service provision in country A
by health professionals who are nationals of country B

---

69. Technological or practical constraints may render some modes of trade unfeasible, for example, cross-border supply (Mode 1) of nursing services. Nevertheless, rapid improvements in telecommunications infrastructure coupled with falling costs have allowed for the supply of services such as medical claims processing and medical records transcription on a cross-border basis.

70. Though data on individuals crossing borders to purchase health services is not collected systematically, consumption abroad (Mode 2) is thought to be growing. Several countries have identified 'health tourism' as an economic development opportunity, whether by providing complex tertiary services at lower cost, bundling health services and marketing them to foreigners, or providing services to returning expatriates (UNCTAD and WHO, 1998).

71. "Commercial presence" (Mode 3) relates to the legal establishment of a foreign service supplier in the territory of the Member concerned. In most cases, foreign investment (FDI) is involved. In turn, such investment tends to be associated with technology transfer; in the health field, this might take the form of modern hospital or health insurance management practices. In several Latin American countries, foreign

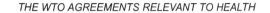

pharmaceutical firms have invested in service providers as part of broader disease management strategies.

72. Presence of natural persons (Mode 4), although accounting for only a limited share in total trade flows, is the most visible of the four modes of supply in health services. The movement of health professionals from less developed to more developed countries is the most prominent example of this mode of health service trade.

(i) GATS general obligations

73. Certain obligations apply across all service sectors, regardless of whether they have been included in a Member's Schedule of Commitments. These unconditional obligations, include most-favored nation treatment (MFN), certain transparency and notification obligations, and certain competition principles.

74. The MFN obligation in GATS requires Members to treat equally services and suppliers of services from all other WTO Members (GATS, Article II). If a Member permits trade in services in a sector, then all suppliers from other Members must be treated on equal terms, regardless of country of ownership or origin. By the same token, any trade restriction must be applied vis-à-vis all other Members. These provisions do not prevent Members from entering into Economic Integration Agreements or recognizing the standards and regulations of one or more trading partners, subject to certain conditions. Furthermore, signatories could have sought exemptions from the MFN obligation at the time the GATS came into effect in 1995, and some 400 such exemptions were listed. In principle, these exemptions should not last more than 10 years; they will be subject to negotiation in any subsequent rounds.

75. Any services supplied in the exercise of governmental authority are excluded from GATS. Article I:3 establishes two criteria defining such services: they must be "supplied neither on a commercial basis, nor in competition with one or more service suppliers". There are some services to which these criteria clearly apply, such as free medical treatment in public facilities Since governmental services do not fall under the Agreement, these services are not covered by the negotiations, and commitments on market access and national treatment do not apply to them. This is a principle to which all Member Governments attach great importance and which none has sought to reopen. So far, Members have not expressed the need to adopt an authoritative inter-

pretation of the criteria in Article I:3(c). They could obviously do so whenever they deem it desirable or appropriate. Also, the issue could arise if a specific measure which had been challenged in dispute settlement proceedings were to be defended on the ground that it applied only to services supplied in the exercise of governmental authority. There is no requirement to notify such services.

76. Under Article XIV of GATS, Members are entitled to take any measure necessary to protect human, animal or plant life or health, regardless of their obligations under the Agreement. The same proviso applies as under Article XX of the GATT: application of a measure must not discriminate arbitrarily or unjustifiably between countries where like conditions prevail, it must not constitute a disguised restriction on trade in services. Like any other trade measure, action under Article XIV may be challenged by affected countries under the WTO dispute settlement mechanism if they feel that the relevant provisions have not been respected.

(ii) Country options for GATS commitments in health services

77. GATS allows WTO Members to choose which service sectors to open up to trade and foreign competition and which modes of service to liberalize. Since GATS, 40 per cent of WTO Members (over 50 countries) have made some type of commitment on health services, compared with 70 per cent on financial and/or telecommunications services. Well over 100 Members have made commitments in financial services, which may have implications for health systems to the extent that health insurance has been included in that context.

78. Sectors in which WTO Members choose to make commitments are inscribed in schedules which also specify any limitations and conditions on market access and national treatment. Moreover, Members may undertake additional commitments concerning any other measures (including standards or qualifications) affecting trade in services.

79. An unqualified market access means the WTO Member agrees not to maintain or adopt measures that restrict the number of service providers, value of service transactions, number of service operators, number of natural persons, types of permissible legal entities, and foreign capital participation. If Members want to reserve the right to operate such restrictions, the relevant measures must be inscribed as limitations to

market access in their Schedules. Members making market access commitments still retain substantial scope for national policy making. For example, a requirement that hospitals devote 25 per cent of beds to care for the uninsured, if applied to all suppliers, does not constitute a market access limitation: it would rather be a matter of domestic regulation. If it were applied only to foreign-owned hospitals, it would still be permitted under GATS provided it was scheduled as a national treatment limitation.

80. In GATS, an unqualified national treatment requires Members to treat all services and service suppliers of any other Member no less favourably than its own like services and service suppliers. However, GATS regards national treatment as a conditional (and negotiable) obligation which may be made subject to conditions or qualifications that Members inscribe in their schedules (GATS Article XVII). Together with the market-access commitments, these conditions or qualifications represent the minimum treatment of a foreign service or supplier to which the country binds itself; countries may offer better treatment in practice.

81. Market access and national treatment commitments must be specified for each mode of supply within each scheduled sector: There are three principal options (i) full commitments, that is commitments without limitations, (ii) limited (or partial) commitments, which are subject to some restrictions or qualifications and (iii) no commitments ("unbound"), where the Member remains free to introduce restrictions on trade in that mode at any time. Commitments must not necessarily be implemented at the end of the negotiations concerned, but can be postponed to a later date specified in the Member's schedule. Such "pre-commitments" provide time for the authorities concerned to undertake any domestic regulatory and institutional changes that may be necessary to ensure compliance.

82. Governments may make commitments for various reasons: to encourage suppliers to enter the market; improve the volume, range and quality of the services available; attract foreign direct investment (FDI) and the related flows of skills and expertise; promote efficiency, and/or stimulate competition in a service sector. As noted elsewhere, the GATS commitments undertaken in the Uruguay Round have served mainly to maintain the status quo regarding market access and national treatment for foreign suppliers. It should be stressed that the absence of a commitment does not mean that trade is prohibited; trade may occur, depending on the regime in place, but foreign suppliers have no guarantee of market access or national treatment.[14]

83. Although a commitment is legally binding, it is not cast in stone. Governments may modify or withdraw it at any time three years after its entry into force. However, where the proposed

---

14. For example, in the context of negotiations on basic telecommunications, concluded in February 1997, a significant number of participating Members undertook to implement their commitments only several years later.

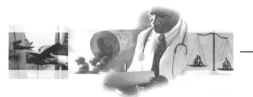

withdrawal or modification affects another country, the country proposing the change may be asked by trading partners to offer equivalent commitments in compensation.

F. SOLVING DISPUTES

84. Formal dispute settlement at the WTO is a last-resort option. As stated in the conclusions of this report, it is preferable that countries should solve their differences among themselves, whether bilaterally, plurilaterally or multilaterally (see paragraph 307). Many differences between Members are unlikely ever to become an issue at the WTO, and even if they do, they will not necessarily trigger formal dispute settlement procedures. Some issues are settled at the committee level or defused in that context. Nevertheless, in the case where two or more Members of the WTO have a dispute over a health-related trade measure and are unable to come to a solution among themselves (or in other fora), they have the right to bring the dispute to the WTO.

85. The WTO Secretariat cannot challenge any Member. It has no right to prosecute. It is up to governments to decide whether or not to bring a dispute against another government to the WTO. And it is also entirely up to the complainant to argue its case. The dispute is only between governments, and only about alleged failures to comply with WTO agreements or commitments. So, for example, a government cannot complain about another government's health policy as such. It can only complain if it believes a particular measure breaks an agreement or commitment that the other government has made in the WTO. Companies, organizations or private individuals cannot complain directly to the WTO, but can do so through their governments.

86. Settling disputes is the responsibility of the Dispute Settlement Body (the "DSB"), which is the WTO General Council in another guise (See above, Chart 1). The DSB has sole authority to establish "panels" of experts to consider the case, and to adopt the panels' findings or the results of an appeal. It monitors the implementation of the rulings and recommendations of panels and the Appellate Body, and has the power to authorise retaliation when a country does not comply with a ruling.

How are disputes settled?

87. One of the most profound changes introduced by the transition from GATT to the WTO in 1995 was the agreement to implement a dispute settlement process that would be speedier and more "automatic", with fixed deadlines (see below, Chart 2). This

Agreement is set out in the WTO Understanding on Rules and Procedures Governing the Settlement of Disputes (the "Dispute Settlement Understanding" or the "DSU"). It is more automatic in the sense that the dispute settlement process, including the adoption of the final panel report and the authorization of sanctions in case of non-compliance, can only be *blocked* if there is a *consensus* to do so (sometimes referred to as "reversed consensus"). Previously, under the GATT, it took a *consensus* among all countries *to adopt* the report - hence the "losing" party to the dispute could always block an unfavourable ruling.

88. In a first stage, the DSU requires countries in dispute to consult with each other to see if they can settle their differences by themselves (for at least 60 days). Parties can also agree to ask the WTO Director-General to mediate. Mediation, conciliation and good offices may be requested at any time in parallel to the dispute settlement process. If the consultations between the parties fail, the complaining country can ask for a panel to be appointed. The country "in the dock" can block the creation of a panel once, but cannot do so when the DSB meets for a second time (unless there is a consensus against appointing the panel).

89. Panels resemble arbitral tribunals, the composition of which is normally also under the control of the parties to the dispute. Only if the two sides cannot agree does the WTO director-general appoint them. Panels consist of three (occasionally five) experts from different countries, who examine the evidence. Panellists for each case can be chosen from a permanent list of qualified candidates, or from elsewhere. They serve in their individual capacities. They cannot receive instructions from any government. Officially, panel and Appellate Body rulings and recommendations "help" the DSB to make its rulings or recommendations. However, because the reports of panels and the Appellate Body can only be rejected by consensus in the DSB, their conclusions are difficult to overturn. Panel and Appellate Body findings have to be based on the agreements cited and should normally be given to the parties to the dispute within nine months from the establishment of the panel.

90. In general, after two hearings with the parties (and technical experts, if necessary)[15], the panel submits the descriptive sections of its report (facts and arguments) for comments to the parties. These do not include any conclusions or findings; the purpose at this stage is to ensure that there is no misunderstanding on the facts of the case. This is followed by an "interim report" also submitted to the parties for review,

---

[15]. If one party raises scientific or other technical matters, the panel may consult experts or appoint an expert review group to prepare an advisory report. In all SPS cases, for example, expert advice was sought.

and then, the final report, which is first submitted to the parties and then later circulated to all WTO Members. Subsequently, the final report is passed to the DSB, which can only reject the report by consensus. The report becomes the DSB's ruling or recommendation within 60 days and is posted on the WTO website.

91. Panel reports can be appealed. The Appellate Body can hear on appeal only points of law decided by panels. Generally, the Appellate Body is not allowed to review facts of the case, as determined by the panel, or examine any evidence. Each appeal is heard by three members of a quasi-permanent seven-member Appellate Body set up by the DSB. Members of the Appellate Body have four-year terms and may be reappointed once. They have to be individuals with recognized standing in the field of law and international trade, and not affiliated with any government. The Appellate Body can uphold, modify or reverse the panel's legal findings and conclusions, and proceedings should normally not last more than 90 days. When a case has been appealed, the DSB has to adopt the reports of the Appellate Body and of the panel (as amended, reversed or upheld) within 30 days from the circulation of the Appellate Body report; rejection is only possible by consensus.

92. The Dispute Settlement Understanding stresses that "prompt compliance with recommendations or rulings of the DSB is essential in order to ensure effective resolution of disputes to the benefit of all Members". If a country is found to be at fault with the rules, it is expected to promptly correct the measure at issue. Moreover, it must state its intention to do so at a DSB meeting held within 30 days of the report's adoption. If immediate compliance with the recommendation proves impractical, the country will be allowed a "reasonable period of time". If it fails to act within this period, it has to enter into negotiations with the complaining country (or countries) in order to determine temporary compensation - for instance, tariff reductions in areas of particular interest to the complaining side. There is no financial compensation. If no satisfactory compensation is agreed, the complaining side may ask the DSB for permission to impose limited trade sanctions ("suspend concessions or obligations") against the other side. If requested the DSB must grant this authorization. WTO Arbitration on the level of such sanctions can also be requested if the parties do not agree.

93. The DSB monitors how adopted rulings are implemented, and any outstanding case remains on its agenda until the issue is resolved. There have been a several disputes relevant to health, a number of which are described in the next Chapter.

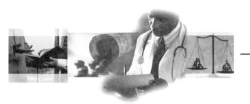

Chart 2: The Panel process

The various stages a dispute can go through in the WTO. At all stages, countries in dispute are encouraged to consult each other in order to settle 'out of court'. At all stages the WTO Director-General is available to offer his good offices, to mediate or to help achieve a conciliation.

NOTE: some specified time periods are maximum, some minimum, some binding, some not.

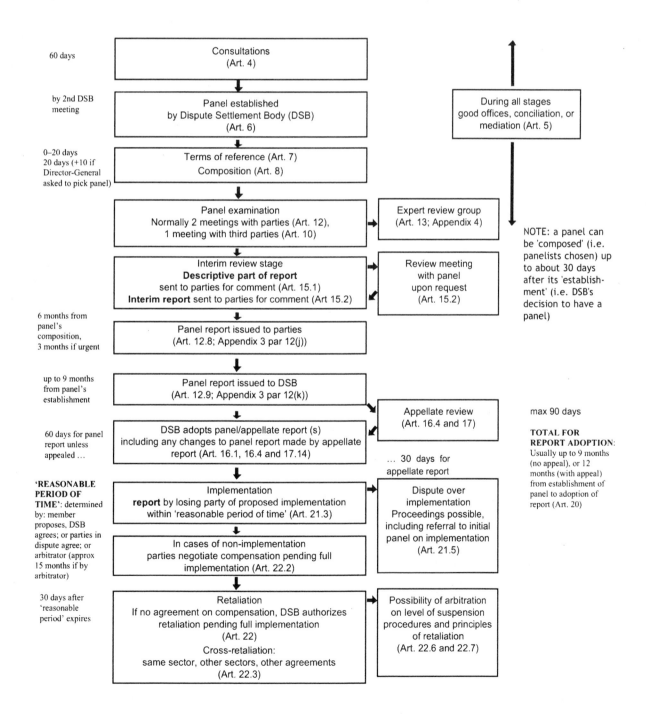

60 days	Consultations (Art. 4)
by 2nd DSB meeting	Panel established by Dispute Settlement Body (DSB) (Art. 6)
0–20 days 20 days (+10 if Director-General asked to pick panel)	Terms of reference (Art. 7) Composition (Art. 8)
	Panel examination Normally 2 meetings with parties (Art. 12), 1 meeting with third parties (Art. 10) → Expert review group (Art. 13; Appendix 4)
	Interim review stage **Descriptive part of report** sent to parties for comment (Art. 15.1) **Interim report** sent to parties for comment (Art 15.2) → Review meeting with panel upon request (Art. 15.2)
6 months from panel's composition, 3 months if urgent	Panel report issued to parties (Art. 12.8; Appendix 3 par 12(j))
up to 9 months from panel's establishment	Panel report issued to DSB (Art. 12.9; Appendix 3 par 12(k)) → Appellate review (Art. 16.4 and 17)
60 days for panel report unless appealed ...	DSB adopts panel/appellate report (s) including any changes to panel report made by appellate report (Art. 16.1, 16.4 and 17.14) ... 30 days for appellate report
'REASONABLE PERIOD OF TIME': determined by: member proposes, DSB agrees; or parties in dispute agree; or arbitrator (approx 15 months if by arbitrator)	Implementation **report** by losing party of proposed implementation within 'reasonable period of time' (Art. 21.3) In cases of non-implementation parties negotiate compensation pending full implementation (Art. 22.2) → Dispute over implementation Proceedings possible, including referral to initial panel on implementation (Art. 21.5)
30 days after 'reasonable period' expires	Retaliation If no agreement on compensation, DSB authorizes retaliation pending full implementation (Art. 22) Cross-retaliation: same sector, other sectors, other agreements (Art. 22.3) → Possibility of arbitration on level of suspension procedures and principles of retaliation (Art. 22.6 and 22.7)

During all stages good offices, conciliation, or mediation (Art. 5)

NOTE: a panel can be 'composed' (i.e. panelists chosen) up to about 30 days after its 'establishment' (i.e. DSB's decision to have a panel)

max 90 days

TOTAL FOR REPORT ADOPTION: Usually up to 9 months (no appeal), or 12 months (with appeal) from establishment of panel to adoption of report (Art. 20)

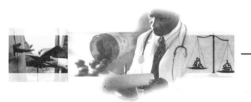

III. SPECIFIC HEALTH ISSUES AND WTO AGREEMENTS

INTRODUCTION

A. INTRODUCTION

94. As noted in the preceding Chapter, several WTO agreements are relevant to health policy. Generally, the positive growth and income effects of more open and predictable trade regimes can provide the resources, as well as goods, services and information, for effective health systems.[16] The WTO agreements explicitly allow governments, in pursuing national health and other policy objectives, to take measures to restrict trade in order to protect health. This is legitimate as a matter of principle. The emphasis in WTO rules is on *how* policies are pursued without questioning the underlying objective. For example, is a measure applied or enforced in a way that discriminates between trading partners or between imported products and products produced domestically? Are there ways of implementing policy that would be less restrictive on trade? Thus, it is the manner in which government pursue specific health policies in practice which might have trade-related implications, which are examined in this Chapter.

95. Putting WTO rules into practice can raise difficult questions for health policy makers. For example, what happens when, for a given hazard, there is uncertainty about the risk? This poses a challenge for regulatory action, and responses to uncertainty and risk are likely to be different in different countries. Among the factors to be considered may be the trade-restrictiveness and efficacy of the measure to achieve the level of health protection sought.

96. This Chapter does not provide definitive answers to these questions. In the end, these are matters for decision-makers in national governments. The discussion of how different countries have addressed such questions sheds light on how health and trade policies can promote synergies in some cases, and how they continue to give rise to tensions in others.

97. The Chapter is organized around eight important health issues facing national policy makers which relate to one or more of the WTO agreements. For each of the eight issues, the trade relevance is explained and applicable WTO agreements are discussed.

[16.] For more information on inputs for effective health systems see WHO World Health Report, 2000.

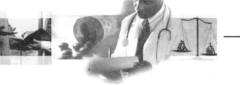

Box 5
Specific health issues and most relevant WTO agreements[1]

WTO Rule or Agreement	Agriculture	SPS	TBT	TRIPS	Services (GATS)	GATT Article XX(b)	Other
Health Issue							
Infectious Disease Control		X	X			X	
Food Safety		X					
Tobacco Control	X		X	X	X	X	
Environment		X	X			X	
Access to Drugs				X			
Health Services					X		X
Food Security	X	X				X	
Emerging Issues							
- Biotechnology	X	X	X	X			
- Information Technology				X	X		
- Traditional Knowledge				X			

1. *Mention is made of only the **most** relevant agreements to the specific health issues.*

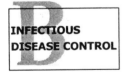

B. INFECTIOUS DISEASE CONTROL

(i) The link between trade and infectious disease control

98. Cross-border movements of people as well as trade in goods and services are increasing the challenges for infectious disease control. The risk of infectious disease rises with increased mobility of people, growth in international trade in food and biological products, and social and environmental changes. These developments affect all elements in the infectious disease chain: hosts (people), agents (microbes causing disease), and vectors (means by which microbes come into contact with people).

99. The variety of transmission methods and the increase in volume of trade of all kinds means that to effectively control disease outbreaks in today's world, public health officials need to collect and disseminate information quickly. Likewise, trade officials who negotiate and implement trade agreements need to be aware of health risks. In most cases, sound public health practice will focus on the mode of transmission-for example, sexual behaviour and drug use in the case of HIV/AIDS - rather than restrict the mobility of people or goods.

(ii) International Health Regulations (IHR) - a global regulatory framework

100. In exceptional circumstances, infectious disease control may require trade or travel restrictions. In the past, disease outbreak control concentrated on quarantines or trade embargoes.[17] In recent years, a combination of sensitive early warning surveillance systems, rapid verification procedures and international response networks, epidemic preparedness plans and stockpiles of essential medicines has reduced the need to employ trade embargoes or travel restrictions. To the extent trade restrictions are used, they should be time-limited and try to minimize disruption to international trade. This is one of the fundamental principles underlying WHO's current revision of the IHR. The renewed IHR will serve as the legal framework for WHO's efforts to prevent disease epidemics from spreading globally. The historic purpose of the IHR is to "ensure the maximum security against the international spread of diseases, with a minimum interference with world traffic." This purpose will continue in the new IHR.

(iii) Trade rules are unlikely to restrict governments' actions to control infectious diseases, but do impose some disciplines ...

101. Specific measures used to control infectious diseases, whether adopted by national governments, or recommended by WHO in the performance of its IHR duties, may be subject to WTO rules if they affect trade in goods or services. Which rules are relevant will depend on the circumstances of the particular case. For example, while sanitary measures to halt the spread of a food-or animal-borne infectious disease could have a substantial trade impact and would be covered by the SPS Agreement, it is unlikely that regulatory action aimed at mitigating such risks - whatever the pathway or nature of the disease - would run contrary to WTO rules.

[17] This is not very far in the past, as witnessed by Peru - cholera, 1991; India - plague, 1994. Most embargoes were avoided during the recent nipah virus and H5N5 outbreaks in Asia by destroying animals.

102. However, much will depend on how this health objective is enforced in practice at the border. WTO rules require, for example, that the measure used should be properly balanced between the importance of the health interests protected, the efficacy of the measure and the impact of the law on imports and exports - to the extent that this is feasible without compromising the intended health objective (see paragraph 23). If it is possible to enforce the health objective through checks or sampling rather than an outright ban, that would be preferable as it is the measure which would least interfere with trade while guaranteeing the level of health protection chosen by that Member. Since quarantines and trade embargoes are associated with substantial economic losses, these restrictions run the risk of being challenged unless they are unquestionably justified by the severity of the health risk. Likewise WTO rules on non-discrimination apply. If a country's sanitary measure addresses a risk in products coming from one country but ignores similar risks in products originating from another country, the measure might be challenged as discriminatory. Such discriminatory action could flag, or serve as a warning signal, that the objective behind the measure at issue may not solely be concerned with protecting health.

Box 6
Safety of imported fish during a cholera outbreak

In early 1998, Tanzania complained in a SPS Committee meeting that the European Communities (EC) was unfairly blocking imports of fish from certain African countries. In response, the EC told the WTO SPS Committee that it had indeed banned imports of fruit, vegetables and fish products in light of a cholera outbreak in Tanzania, Kenya, Uganda and Mozambique. EC inspection procedures in these countries had uncovered deficiencies, and the EC sought to put in effect proper hygiene requirements. EC Member States, meanwhile, were trying to develop a joint cholera policy based on risk assessment.

A WHO investigator had told the EC that she did not consider the ban on fish imports necessary, since fish products were not consumed in raw form in Europe. She cited the WHO Guidance on Formulation of National Policy on the Control of Cholera: "Although there is a theoretical risk of cholera transmission associated with some food commodities moving in international trade, this has rarely proved significant and authorities should seek means of dealing with it other than by applying an embargo on importation".

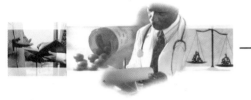

**Box 6
Safety of imported fish during a cholera outbreak (cont'd)**

In June 1998, Tanzania reported to the SPS Committee that the EC continued to prohibit the importation of fresh, frozen and processed fishery products from the four African countries, although tests had not found the bacteria concerned. Tanzania stressed that the EC ban was having severe effects on its economy. After a WHO official attested again - this time to the SPS Committee - that there was no proven risk of cholera transmission from the foods in question, and after an EU Scientific Committee reiterated this statement, the European Communities agreed to resume trade on 1 July 1998. The case underscores the importance of basing trade-restrictive public health measures on scientific evidence, rather than theoretical risk. It also demonstrates the usefulness to the SPS Committee of WHO recommendations based on the specific health risks of each situation.

(iv) Revising the IHR to cope with new threats to health

103. Cholera is a long-standing, endemic disease with well-known control measures. But the modern era has witnessed the emergence of new global health security threats, for which control measures are still evolving. HIV/AIDS was unknown until about 20 years ago and new pathogens have come to light, such as the Ebola and Marburg viruses. In addition, many "older" diseases (such as tuberculosis, malaria and sexually transmitted diseases) have become a greater threat because they have developed resistance to the drugs commonly used to treat them.[18]

104. These developments prompted WHO in 1995 to call for a revision of the IHR. It had become less useful as a tool to control the global spread of disease for several reasons. IHR covers only plague, cholera and yellow fever, while global health security can be threatened by a far wider set of diseases and infectious agents. In addition, the IHR "maximum measures" for control needed to be more flexible to tailor solutions to the particular circumstances surrounding each risk. Furthermore, IHR contains no enforcement provisions nor does it have any incentives to promote adherence to its recommendations and depends on the willingness of countries to make official notifications to WHO, which they have little incentive to do given the potential economic costs.

---

18. There have been other recent outbreaks relevant to trade, such as the H5N5 outbreak in Hong Kong (poultry, fowl), nipah virus in Malaysia (pigs), rift valley fever (cattle) in Ethiopia. All of these diseases "crossed over" to humans.

105. Revision of the IHR will focus on three areas. One involves expansion of the scope of notifications required of Member States, to cover *public health emergencies of international concern*. Member States would be required to notify WHO of all such emergencies that occur in their territory. A specific algorithm, or tool, is being developed to help countries assess the potential importance and urgency of such an event in collaboration with WHO, to determine if a public health emergency exists. Second, WHO will attempt to strengthen IHR by using information from other reliable sources (besides official ones) to identify new outbreaks, for example through greater reliance on WHO's global outbreak alert and verification process. Third, WHO will seek ways of making its recommendations for control measures, issued at the time of a public health emergency, consistent with WTO Member rights and obligations under the SPS Agreement. Most of the outbreaks that will be addressed by the IHR will involve disease transmission through person-to-person spread, rather than through traded goods such as foodstuffs.

106. Several challenges remain in the IHR revision process. Efforts must be made to ensure that only public health risks (usually those caused by an infectious agent) that are of urgent international importance are reported, while devising a system sensitive enough to pick up new or re-emerging public health risks. Steps must also be taken to avoid stigmatization and unnecessary negative impact on international travel and trade caused by invalid reporting from sources other than Member States, which can have serious economic consequences for countries. If the proposed IHR contains a list of measures that could restrict the free movement of people, conveyances and goods during public health emergencies, it is important that they are properly "aimed" when used. In addition, because trade can be adversely affected when certain public health risks occur, the revised IHR must reflect a consensus among health and trade interests, requiring close consultation between officials at the national level, and between WHO and the WTO at the international level. The target date for submission of the revised IHR to the World Health Assembly is May 2004.

C. FOOD SAFETY

(i) Global incidence of food-borne disease...

107. WHO estimates that world-wide almost 2 million children die every year from diarrhoea, most of this caused by microbiologically contaminated food and water (WHO, 1999a). Even in industrialized countries it is estimated that one third of the population

suffers from food-borne disease every year, and out of these maybe up to 20 per million die. Considering that these figures only relate to microbiological problems, the addition of chemical contamination of food makes the situation extremely serious. The epidemic nature of outbreaks of food-borne disease varies from localised and self-limiting out-breaks - which would not be relevant to international trade - to rapidly spreading epidemics that can quickly cross international borders via trade.[19]

(ii) ... and the link to trade

108. Several new sources of food-borne illness are of increasing relevance to international trade. In the past few years, chemical hazards in food-related products have been the source of several limited, but highly publicized health crises, for example the contamination of animal feed by dioxin in Belgium that affected food products throughout Europe. Changing patterns of farming and animal husbandry can also affect food safety, illustrated by the spread of mad cow disease (BSE) and its onward transmission to people which manifests as vCJD, a fatal neurological disease. The widespread use of antibiotics in animal husbandry has contributed to increased levels of antibiotic-resistant bacteria in humans. In addition, the safety for human consumption of certain genetically modified foods is a matter of concern to some.

109. All of these food safety concerns come into play in the context of international trade in foods, which has grown substantially over the past 10 years. Agriculture and food exports are essential to most developing countries as many have a comparative advantage in agricultural production. Furthermore, the trend towards the export of more and more processed foods is increasing the importance of sanitary and phytosanitary measures and the SPS Agreement.[20] Also, as was noted in Chapter II, as tariffs and other classical barriers to trade are likely to fall further in the context of further agricultural reform - including support to agricultural production in the richer countries - the relative importance of non-tariff measures is likely to increase.

[19]. A big burden of food-borne disease also lies in the sporadic cases, which are not linked to outbreaks, and therefore typically are not recognized or reported.

[20]. World Bank, "The Development Challenge in Trade: Sanitary and Phytosanitary Standards", Submission by the World Bank to the WTO SPS Committee, 12 July 2000, G/SPS/GEN/195.

Box 7
SPS and Codex[1]

The Joint Food and Agriculture Organization/World Health Organization (FAO/WHO) Codex Alimentarius Commission (Codex) was established in 1962 to establish standards for food safety. The Commission currently has 165 member governments who, with the advice of independent technical experts selected by FAO and WHO, develop food standards, guidelines and recommendations for the protection of consumer health. Codex recognizes the importance of minimizing the effect of such regulations on food trade. Member states formally endorse Codex standards, after thorough reviews of scientific papers based on widely accepted risk assessment procedures. While it remains voluntary for governments to apply Codex standards, there are strong incentives to do so, as food production that meets Codex standards can facilitate trade by creating greater export opportunities.

Many new ideas are being integrated into Codex recommendations and standards. Codex now recommends using a risk-based preventive approach in achieving food safety, and promotes the use of formalized Risk analysis. An example of a approach is the implementation of the Hazard Analysis and Critical Control Point (HACCP) system. HACCP encourages the food industry and governments to target limited resources to the most critical steps of food production and distribution, rather than having to comply with a long list of product and procedure specifications as has been traditionally prescribed. HACCP often requires reorientation of food safety authorities towards audit and training functions, rather than on physical inspection and laboratory analysis. Although HACCP does not completely eliminate the necessity for final product inspection, the concept of process control is central to HACCP national food safety programmes.

Another important trend in Codex is its horizontal approach. Codex is in the process of elaborating general standards covering food additives, contaminants and toxins to provide a wider basis for protecting consumers' health. Countries can better adapt themselves to this approach by implementing a generic regulation applicable to a wide range of products rather than maintaining an inventory of registered foods with specifications for each.

[1]. *For further information about food safety and trade issues, see the WHO publication, Food Safety and Globalization of Trade in Food, 1998 (revised), visit WHO's website on Food Safety: http://www.who.int/fsf, or go directly to the Codex website: http://www.fao.org/es/esn/codex/*

(iii) The SPS Agreement is perhaps the closest "match" between a health issue (in this case food safety) and trade

110. Unlike some other "health issues" in this report, food safety has one WTO Agreement which is specifically relevant: the SPS Agreement (for an overview see pages 34-38). It applies to any trade-related measure taken to protect human life or health from risks arising from additives, contaminants, toxins, veterinary drug and pesticide residues, or other disease-causing organisms in foods or beverages. The SPS Agreement clearly gives governments the right to restrict trade to achieve health objectives, but the measures applied must be based on scientific evidence.

111. The SPS Agreement formally recognizes the food safety standards, guidelines and recommendations established by the FAO/WHO Codex Alimentarius Commission (Codex for short). The recognition of Codex standards eliminates the need for each country individually to do its own risk assessment for any given hazard for which a standard, recommendation or guideline exists. If countries adopt national food safety standards that are not more stringent than the Codex standards, and have mechanisms for monitoring compliance among food producers and exporters with these standards, then their food safety measures are presumed to be consistent with SPS provisions. Recognizing that many global food safety issues lie beyond the reach of international trade agreements, WHO together with FAO and national governments are stepping up efforts to ensure that consumers across the globe are protected from threats to food safety from a wide range of sources.

(iv) How is the WTO "used" to address food safety concerns?

112. Since the WTO SPS Agreement came into force in 1995, more than 100 specific trade concerns have been raised in the SPS Committee, of which about 30 are directly relevant to food safety. The remaining trade concerns have dealt with animal and plant health issues which are equally relevant to the SPS Agreement. The food safety issues range from discussions on restrictions on imports of hard cheeses made from non-pasteurised milk to labelling requirements on shelled eggs, or shelf-life requirements for canned food products.

113. The number of specific trade concerns related to food safety is not limited to issues actually raised in the SPS Committee. Many concerns regarding food safety meas-

ures are solved bilaterally before they come to the WTO, or around the edges of the SPS Committee meetings without actually having been raised at the meeting itself. Whether raising an issue in the SPS Committee is the most effective way to address the problem is for the government concerned to decide. Nevertheless, a key function of the SPS Committee is that of a forum where any country can raise any issue related to food safety and trade, and in the past a number of useful decisions have been adopted by the SPS Committee.

114. Only one issue relevant to human health, trade and food safety has gone through the entire dispute settlement process. This is the so-called EC-Hormones dispute between the United States, Canada and the European Union. Like the cholera case, the beef hormone case underscores the importance of basing food safety regulations on scientific evidence and international food safety standards.

Box 8
"EC - Hormones"
WTO panel on European Community -
measures concerning meat and meat products (hormones),
complaints by the United States and Canada[1]

The case grew out of suggestions related to known and unknown effects of hormones and European consumers' concern over the use of hormones for growth promotion purposes in livestock, a practice that grew steadily throughout the 1970s. The WHO-FAO Joint Expert Committee on Food Additives (JECFA) examined the use of these hormones and their health implications. On the basis of the JECFA recommendations, the Codex adopted standards for five of the growth-promoting hormones. The standards specified the maximum level of hormone residues in foods that are safe for human consumption. Despite these standards, several scandals concerning the use of illegal hormonal substances prompted the European Union in 1988 to completely ban the use of growth-promoting hormones. In January 1996, the US, followed by Canada in June of the same year, challenged this EU decision as inconsistent with the SPS Agreement.

In 1998, the Appellate Body ruled that the EC was in violation of SPS rules. As the international Codex standards existed for five of the six hormones at issue, the panel judged that the EC was required to justify its ban, and hence its non-application of the international standards, on the basis of its own assessment of the risks to human health. The scientific evidence presented by the EU did not support the ban on hormones. The WTO Appellate Body affirmed the decision of the panel that the EC ban was in violation of the SPS Agreement because it was not based on a risk assessment.

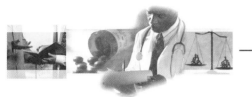

Box 8
"EC - Hormones"
WTO panel on European Community -
Measures concerning meat and meat products (hormones),
complaints by the United States and Canada[1] (cont'd)

But the Appellate Body also confirmed the rights of Members to have the level of health protection they want, even above international standards, and that it is for the Member challenging an SPS measure to bear the burden of proof. In May 1998, an arbitrator gave the EC until 13 May 1999 to implement the recommendations of the Dispute Settlement Body. As the EC was unable to act accordingly and failed to lift its import ban, on 12 July 1999, the WTO authorized the United States and Canada to impose compensatory measures in the form of the suspension of tariff concessions covering trade to a maximum amount of $US 116.8 million per year for the United States and CDN$ 11.3 million per year for Canada. These measures are still in force.

[1]. *WTO Symbol: WT/DS26/R/USA and WT/DS48/R/CAN, dated 18 August 1997 and the Appellate Report WT/DS26/AB/R, WT/DS48/AB/R, dated 16 January 1998.*

(v) The use of "precaution" in food safety

115. What happens, however, when scientific evidence is inconclusive regarding possible risks to human health from certain types of foods? There may be cases where the lack of conclusive scientific evidence about risks to health and the environment do not justify regulatory inaction. According to Article 5.7 of the SPS Agreement, provisional measures are allowed in the absence of sufficient scientific evidence.

Box 9
Article 5.7 of the SPS Agreement

"In cases where relevant scientific evidence is insufficient, a Member may provisionally adopt sanitary or phytosanitary measures on the basis of available pertinent information, including that from the relevant international organizations as well as from sanitary or phytosanitary measures applied by other Members. In such circumstances, Members shall seek to obtain the additional information necessary for a more objective assessment of risk and review the sanitary or phytosanitary measure accordingly within a reasonable period of time."

116. In the EC-Hormones case, the EC did not invoke Article 5.7 of the SPS Agreement. Rather, the EC attempted to justify its hormones ban by arguing that the "precautionary principle" was a general principle under international law. In other words, the EC invoked the "precautionary principle" in general terms as an overriding principle, while never claiming that the ban on imports of hormone-treated meat was in any way "provisional". The Appellate Body noted that the "precautionary principle", other than as reflected in Article 5.7, did not override the obligation to *base SPS measures on a risk assessment*.

117. The only directly relevant jurisprudence on Article 5.7 of the SPS Agreement is from the *Japan-Varietals* case.[21] In this case, the Panel found that the testing requirement imposed by Japan on certain fruit products could not be considered as a provisional phytosanitary measure in an area where scientific information was insufficient, since Japan had not sought to obtain the information necessary for a more objective assessment of risk and reviewed the measure accordingly within a reasonable period of time. The AB upheld this finding, and commented on the notion of "reasonable period of time":

"In our view, what constitutes a "reasonable period of time" has to be established on a case-by-case basis and depends on the specific circumstances of each case, including the difficulty of obtaining the additional information necessary for the review and the characteristics of the provisional SPS measure." [22]

118. Japan subsequently notified to the WTO that it had completed technical consultations regarding a new methodology on the products at issue in the dispute and currently subject to the import prohibition and expected shortly to notify the WTO of a "mutually satisfactory solution".[23]

(vi) Challenges for the future

119. While the SPS Agreement and Codex standards have proven to be helpful in resolving several international controversies over the safety of traded foods, there remain significant challenges. Many developing countries have found that for their exports to meet international food safety and quality standards, they need to invest substantially in both physical and institutional infrastructure. Article 9 of the SPS

---

[21]. Japan - Measures Affecting Agricultural Products, Report of the Panel, WT/DS76/R, 27 October 1998 and Report of the Appellate Body, WT/DS76/AB/R, dated 22 February 1999.

[22]. Japan - Measures Affecting Agricultural Products, Report of the Appellate Body, WT/DS76/AB/R, dated 22 February 1999, paragraph 93.

[23]. This information is contained in a "Status Report by Japan" notified to the DSB on 8 June 2001 (WT/DS76/11/Add.5).

Agreement requires developing countries be provided with technical assistance to do this, but there is still a big gap between what is needed and what is provided. In addition, many of the least-developed countries lack the data as well as the capacity and technical expertise to fully participate in Codex standard-setting processes as well as other fora relevant to food safety and or quality issues (WHO, ISO). The funding for developing countries' participation in Codex work is also a problem. Both the WHO and FAO, among other groups, are providing more technical assistance to alleviate this problem, and more Codex meetings take place in each region to make it easier for developing countries to send representatives. Pursuant to a resolution passed by the World Health Assembly in 2000 (WHA 53.15), WHO is also stepping up efforts to support capacity-building in developing countries for critical food safety activities.

120. In an effort to address the problem of effective participation by developing countries in the standard-setting process, an interagency cooperation and coordination mechanism, involving the WTO, the FAO, WHO, OIE (the world animal health organization) and the World Bank, was established to identify ways of facilitating developing country participation in standard-setting activities and addressing their technical assistance needs. In a joint statement delivered at the Doha Ministerial Conference, these organizations affirmed their commitment to "enhance developing countries' capacity to participate effectively in the development and application of international standards and to take full advantage of trade opportunities". A workshop on the development of international standards was held at the WTO in March 2001 to provide information on their respective standard-setting processes, with a focus on maximizing developing country involvement.[24] Since the establishment of the interagency mechanism, several meetings have taken place, and the cooperation of the WTO, the FAO, WHO, OIE and World Bank is ongoing.

(vii) Safety of Genetically Modified Products (GMOs)

121. Another significant challenge on the international food safety agenda concerns new foods derived from genetic modification. The application of biotechnology to food has made food production more efficient in some cases and contributed to increased harvests. It also holds promise for improving public health. For example, "Golden Rice", a genetically modified rice that produces beta-carotene which the body converts into vitamin A, may help to alleviate vitamin A deficiency, a major cause of blindness in developing countries. On the other hand, there are several concerns about the long-

---

24. A summary report of this workshop is contained in G/SPS/GEN/250, available on the WTO website (www.wto.org).

term health effects of genetically-modified (GM) foods, such as: the potential for gene transfer from GM plants to microbial or mammalian cells; the transfer and expression of a functional antibiotic resistance gene to recipient cells in people or animals; and allergenic effects.

122. Reflecting growing concern about the safety and nutritional aspects of foods derived from biotechnology, the Codex Alimentarius Commission decided in July 1999 to undertake "the consideration of standards, guidelines or other recommendations for foods derived from biotechnology or traits introduced into foods by biotechnology." The same session also established an Intergovernmental Task Force on Foods Derived from Biotechnology, with a three-year mandate, to help formulate a global consensus on the safety and nutritional aspects of foods derived from biotechnology. At its March 2002 meeting, the Task Force reached agreement on a final draft of "Principles for the risk analysis of foods derived from biotechnology," which will provide the necessary frame-work for evaluating the safety and nutritional aspects of GM foods. The task force also adopted detailed requirements for assessing the safety of GM plants including tests for allergenicity. In April 2001, FAO and WHO published new recommendations to strength-en the process used to protect consumers from the risk that some GMOs could pose for a small percentage of people with food allergies.[25] Moreover, the July 2001 meeting of the Codex Alimentarius Commission adopted a draft amendment on the labelling of allergens in food or food ingredients obtained through biotechnology.[26]

123. Other challenges lie ahead, particularly the need to develop global standards for pre-market approval systems of genetically modified food to ensure that these new prod-ucts are not only safe, but also beneficial for consumers. On the trade side, arguments are brewing over the feasibility of regulations that would place "traceability" and labelling requirements on bio-engineered foods, and their consistency with WTO trade rules.

---

[25] Evaluation of Allergenicity of Genetically Modified Foods, Report of a Joint FAO/WHO Expert Consultation on Allergenicity of Foods Derived from Biotechnology, 22-25 January 2001.

[26] The adopted amendment is contained in Codex document: Alinorm 01/22 (Appendix 3), p 47. The report of the Codex Alimentarius Commission meeting of July 2001 where this adoption will be reflected, had not yet been posted on the Codex web site (http://www.codexali-mentarius.net/) at the time of writing.

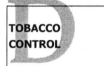

D. TOBACCO CONTROL

(i) The threat

124. Since about 1950, more than 70,000 scientific studies have proven that smoking causes disease, disability and death.[27] About one in every two long-term smokers die from their habit. Tobacco use is a major cause of cardiovascular disease, while 90 per cent of all lung cancers and 75 per cent of all cases of chronic bronchitis and emphysema are due to tobacco. WHO estimates that tobacco products currently kill 4.2 million people each year. By the year 2030 this annual toll will rise to nearly ten million deaths, about 70 per cent of which will occur in developing countries. In other words, tobacco will cause 150 million deaths in the first quarter of the century, and 300 million in the second quarter - if current trends continue. In developed countries, about half of these deaths will occur in people in their most economically productive years. Exposure to cigarette smoke causes higher risk of lung cancer and several other children's health problems - sudden infant death syndrome, low birth weight, and respiratory disease.

(ii) Openness to trade may increase consumption of tobacco

125. Tobacco promotion and trade has become a major global public health threat (Yach and Bettcher, 1998).[28] While tobacco consumption fell in many high-income countries in the 1980s and 1990s, it rose in developing countries. That is largely due to the inroads made by transnational tobacco companies (TTCs) into the markets of poor and middle income nations in the last decade (Jha and Chaloupka, 2000)[29]. TTCs have been strong proponents of tariff reduction and open markets to enable them to compete with domestically manufactured tobacco products in high growth markets in Latin America, Eastern Europe, and Asia. Eliminating or reducing tariffs and other barriers to imported tobacco products enables foreign companies to compete more fairly with locally produced ones. The increase in competition associated with opening the market to foreign producers may also lead to more intensive promotion and marketing of tobacco products.

126. Empirical evidence confirms that trade openness leads to increased tobacco consumption (Taylor, et al., 2000)[30]. Aggressive marketing efforts by TTCs undertaken in the

27. US Department of Health and Human Services. Preventing Tobacco Use Among Young People: A Report of the Surgeon General. US Department of Health and Human Services, Centers for Disease Control, National Center for Chronic Disease Prevention and Health Promotion, Office on Smoking and Health. Washington: US Government Printing Office, 1994.

28. Yach, D., Bettcher, D. The Globalization of Public Health, II: The Convergence of Self Interest and Altruism. AM J Public Health. 1998 May; 88 (5): 738-41; discussion 742-4.

29. Jha, P., Chaloupka, F.J. (eds.) Tobacco Control in Developing Countries. New York: Oxford University Press, 2000.

30. Taylor, A.L., Bettcher, D.W. WHO Framework Convention on Tobacco Control: a Global "Good" for Public Health. Bulletin World Health Organization 2000; 78(7): 920-9. Review.

wake of bilateral agreements negotiated between the USA and several Asian countries in the 1980s stimulated demand for tobacco in an initial period. The evidence also indicates that the effect of TTC marketing on increasing tobacco consumption is greater in the poorer and more vulnerable countries (World Bank, 1999, Taylor, et al., 2000).[31]

(iii) Tobacco control policies

127. What is the economic rationale for intervention in the tobacco market? Economic theory suggests that if consumers know all the risks and bear all the costs of their choices, governments have no reason on efficiency grounds to intervene in a market. But the tobacco market is characterized by several market failures and inefficiencies which necessitate government intervention. These include (i) inadequate information about the health risks of tobacco; (ii) inadequate information about the risks of addiction; and (iii) the physical and financial costs imposed on non-smokers (Jha and Chaloupka, 2000).

128. Studies have documented a range of effective tobacco control policies and interventions that substantially reduce tobacco prevalence and consumption. Studies of the individual and combined effects of various policies showed that increasing the price of tobacco products through excise taxes or duty tariffs constitutes by far the most important policy tool available (Townsend, 1988;[32] Jha and Chaloupka, 2000). Tobacco tax increases that raise the price of cigarettes by at least 10 per cent have been very effective in lowering tobacco use, particularly in developing countries (Jha and Chaloupka, 2000). Non-discriminatory taxation is consistent with WTO rules.

129. Higher tariffs on tobacco may, among other factors (such as taxes), contribute to a rise in consumer price, which leads to lower levels of consumption and lower prevalence of smoking among youth (World Bank, 1999). Raising tariffs, however, runs counter to the general goal of trade liberalization, which is to reduce or eliminate tariffs and non-tariff barriers to international trade. Commitments to reduce tariffs on tobacco products are now part of existing multilateral, regional and bilateral trade agreements. But one of the key objectives of the WTO agreements - reducing tariffs and eliminating non-tariff barriers to trade - does not prevent governments applying non-discriminatory internal taxes and certain other measures which they may consider appropriate to safeguard public health.

[31.] The World Bank. Curbing the Epidemic: Governments and the Economics of Tobacco Control. Series: Development in Practice. Washington DC: The World Bank, 1999.

[32.] Townsend, J. Price, Tax and Smoking in Europe. Copenhagen: World Health Organization, 1998.

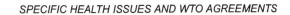
(iv) Tobacco dispute: an example of the application of trade rules

130. The health and tobacco trade debate dates back to the late 1980s. At that time, the US government began a series of actions to get Thailand and some other Asian countries to open their markets to US tobacco products. In each case, tobacco manufacture and sales were controlled by state monopolies. The US government succeeded in negotiating bilateral agreements that removed excise taxes and distribution practices that discriminated against US tobacco products - except in Thailand.

131. Thailand argued that its import restrictions were part of a comprehensive policy to control tobacco use. In response, the United States filed a complaint with the General Agreement on Trade and Tariffs (GATT), the predecessor to the WTO, against Thailand (Box 10). In brief, as a result of this case Thailand had to lift its import ban and reduce the excise duty on tobacco because these could not be justified on health grounds so long as the sale of domestic cigarettes was allowed. But Thailand was allowed to continue with its advertising ban since this applied to all products without discrimination. In line with the GATT ruling, the Thai government lifted the import ban in 1990 and legal exports of cigarettes commenced to Thailand in 1991. Thailand was, of course, still free to charge duty on imports. It was also free to set its excise duty at any level so long as it did not discriminate between local and imported products.

132. The opening of the domestic market to foreign producers initially led to an increase in cigarette consumption, but it also served to strengthen national tobacco control efforts. After the GATT ruling, support grew for national tobacco control measures and in 1992 the Thai parliament passed two important tobacco control acts designed to restrict tobacco sales. The measures included increased sales taxes, smoking bans in public buildings, disclosure of ingredients, and requirements for prominent health warnings on cigarette packages. As a result, smoking prevalence declined in the mid and late 1990s.

133. Most countries, however, face strong challenges to implementing effective, comprehensive tobacco control measures. There is often fierce political opposition from domestic producers, who may be fully or partly owned by the government. Meanwhile, foreign producers continue to seek market access. These challenges are further compounded by international tobacco smuggling.

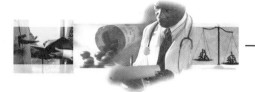

Box 10
WTO dispute: Thailand-Cigarette Case

Under the 1966 Tobacco Act, Thailand prohibited the importation of cigarettes and other tobacco preparations, but authorized the sale of domestic cigarettes. Cigarettes were also made subject to an excise tax, a business tax and a municipal tax. In 1989, The United States complained that the import restrictions were inconsistent with GATT Article XI (on the "General Elimination of Quantitative Restrictions"), and considered that they could not be justified by either (i) some of the exceptions to the elimination of quantitative restrictions allowed for under that same Article, or (ii) Article XX(b) (on "General Exceptions" pertaining to measures necessary for the protection of human life or health). It also argued that the internal taxes were inconsistent with GATT Article III:2 (on "National Treatment on Internal Taxation and Regulation").

Thailand responded by arguing, inter alia, that the import restrictions were justified under Article XX(b) because the government had adopted measures which could only be effective if cigarette imports were prohibited, and because chemicals and other additives contained in United States cigarettes might make them more harmful to human health than Thai cigarettes.

WHO submissions to the GATT dispute panel confirmed differences between cigarettes manufactured in developing countries like Thailand and those in developed countries, which contained more additives and flavouring to make them easier to smoke, especially by women and adolescents. However, WHO did not find any scientific evidence to show that one type of cigarette was more harmful to health than the other.

The Panel found that the import restrictions were inconsistent with Article XI and not justified under the exceptions which that Article allows for. It further concluded that the import restrictions were not "necessary" within the meaning of Article XX(b) (i.e. not necessary for the protection of human life or health). The internal taxes, on the other hand, were found to be consistent with Article III:2.

Import restrictions were found not to be necessary because other methods could be used to protect public health, including various tobacco-control measures, without favouring domestic production. Two of these were bans on advertising and point-of-sale promotion, which applied to cigarettes of all sources. For this reason, the panel rejected the United States call for the advertising ban to be lifted. Thai health and trade officials welcomed this last decision.

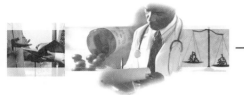

Box 10
WTO Dispute: Thailand-Cigarette Case[1] (cont'd)

Some of these officials said it showed that the GATT dispute settlement process allowed them to defend the advertising ban, whereas countries that had negotiated a settlement bilaterally with the United States outside the GATT had ended up allowing advertising. ("GATT negotiators losing fight against cigarettes" in The Nation, page B4, Bangkok, December 9, 1990).

[1]. This case was brought under the GATT dispute-settlement system before it was revised with the WTO's creation in 1995. The GATT rules cited were also pre-1995. Dispute symbol: DS10/R - 37S/200.

(v) Links between WTO Agreements and Tobacco Policies

134. A growing number of countries have comprehensive tobacco control programs. In addition to tax increases and other price measures, these programs include policies to ban or severely restrict tobacco advertising, expand public health information campaigns, restrict sales through vending machines, ban smoking in public places and encourage cessation of tobacco use, and support for tobacco control coalitions (WHO 1999a)[33]. Depending on how governments choose to manage trade in tobacco and tobacco products, a number of WTO rules could come into play. The US-Thai tobacco case illustrated the relevance of the General Agreement on Tariffs and Trade (GATT), as it affected taxes, prohibitions, and human-health related exceptions to GATT rules. Other WTO agreements that may be applicable, but which have not yet been involved in tobacco-related controversy among WTO Members, include:

(a) the Technical Barriers to Trade (TBT) Agreement in relation to product requirements such as packaging and labelling;
(b) the Agreement on Agriculture in relation to government support for tobacco production;
(c) the General Agreement on Trade in Services (GATS) in relation to restrictions on cigarette advertising; and

[33]. World Health Report 1999 Chapter 5.

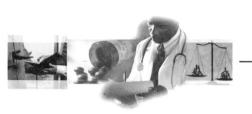
(d) the Agreement on the Trade-Related Aspects of Intellectual Property Rights (TRIPS) in relation to trademark protection and the disclosure of product information considered by producers to be confidential.

(vi) Framework Convention on Tobacco Control - a new international health treaty

135. The challenges to comprehensive tobacco control policies that lie outside national borders led WHO in 1996 to propose the development of a Framework Convention on Tobacco Control (FCTC). Its purpose is to facilitate multilateral cooperation and action at the global level to address transnational tobacco control strategies, the effectiveness of which in reducing demand for tobacco, is substantiated by overwhelming empirical evidence. These include tobacco taxes and prices, restrictions on advertising and promotion, use of mass media and counter-advertising, design of warning labels and packaging, clean indoor air policies, and treatment of tobacco dependence (Taylor and Bettcher, 2000).

136. The Framework Convention calls for cooperation amongst countries in achieving broadly stated goals, and establishes the general norms and institutions of a multilateral legal structure. An accompanying set of protocols will elaborate additional and more specific commitments and institutional arrangements to achieve the goals. WHO Member States began the FCTC negotiation process in October 2000 at the first session of the Intergovernmental Negotiating Body. A second session was held in early May 2001 and the third in November 2001.

137. At the FCTC negotiating sessions, there has been discussion of certain trade-related provisions in the proposed Chairman's text. These provisions include those designed to combat illegal trade and smuggling, phase out duty-free sales and increase and harmonize taxes internationally; and various packaging and labelling issues, such as bans on the use of labels like "low tar" or "mild," which are criticized for giving smokers a false sense of security. Some countries proposed that tobacco products be exempt from reduced tariffs under regional trade agreements. Advertising limits may also have implications vis-à-vis trade agreements.

138. The draft text proposes as a guiding principle that: "Tobacco-control measures should not constitute a means of arbitrary or unjustifiable discrimination in international trade."[34] None of the provisions of the FCTC are inherently WTO-inconsistent; and

---

34. See document at: http://www.who.int/wha-1998/Tobacco/INB2/anglaisINB2.htm

many of the restrictions called for by some of its provisions may well be determined to be "necessary" for health protection under WTO rules. However, some governments and NGOs are arguing that health objectives should take precedence over trade agreements. Thus, the relationship between WTO rules and the FCTC will depend on the direction that future negotiations of the FCTC take, and the manner in which its rules are applied by governments.

(vii) The FCTC negotiations are a good example of the need for international cooperation

139. In the past, several of the potential inconsistencies between Multilateral Environmental Agreements (MEAs) and WTO rules may have arisen as a result of the lack of proper coordination between trade and environment officials both at the national and international levels. In this sense, it is noteworthy that the draft FCTC has been modelled on a number of multilateral agreements, several of which are MEAs. As the relationship between WTO rules and those of other international treaties can offer lessons for the FCTC, WHO intends to monitor the deliberations of the WTO Committee on Trade and Environment where such issues are discussed (next sub-section to the report).

140. A conclusion that can be drawn is that proper coordination between trade and health officials at the national and international levels is crucial to negotiating a WTO-consistent FCTC. In this sense the initiative by the WHO to create the Inter-Agency Task-Force on Tobacco Control for greater coordination between all relevant organizations at an early stage in the negotiations is useful. The WTO, which has observer status in the WHO, follows the negotiations of the FCTC and is part of this Task Force.

E. ENVIRONMENT

(i) The link between environment, health and trade

141. The link between environment and health is well established: most environmental hazards will affect human health in varying degrees. The link between environment, health *and trade* is not as obvious. Economic growth is not sustainable in the long-term if it comes at the expense of the environment, that is, the air, land and water on which human life and health depends. As freer trade has a catalytic effect on growth, *how* such growth takes place becomes more important. In the Preamble to the Marrakesh

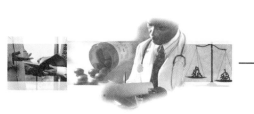

Agreement Establishing the WTO, governments affirmed the importance of working towards sustainable development. The very first paragraph of the Preamble states that WTO Members recognize that their trade and economic relations should be conducted, inter alia,

"... while allowing for the optimal use of the world's resources in accordance with the objective of sustainable development, seeking both to protect and preserve the environment and to enhance the means for doing so in a manner consistent with their respective needs and concerns at different levels of economic development"

142. In the Doha Ministerial Declaration, Ministers strongly reaffirmed their commitment to the objective of sustainable development. They also recognized that, under WTO rules, countries should not be prevented from taking measures for the protection of human, animal or plant life or health, or of the environment at the levels it considers appropriate, subject to the requirement, inter alia, that such measures not be discriminatory.

143. In addressing the link between trade and environment, governments do not operate on the assumption that trade rules are an answer to environmental problems. However, trade and environmental policies can complement each other: environmental protection contributes to the preservation of the natural resource base on which economic growth is premised. From the point of view of developing countries, where poverty is a major concern and an important obstacle to environmental protection, the opening up of world markets to their exports can be part of the solution. Trade liberalization for developing country exports, along with financial and technology transfers, may help developing countries generate resources to protect the environment and work towards sustainable development.

144. For example, in many developing countries, foreign investment can introduce modern equipment and production processes that are safer and less polluting than those used previously. Removing trade barriers to modern "green" technologies and to suppliers of environmental goods and services offers the potential to improve environmental health conditions. The removal of trade distorting policies such as subsidies may both enhance trade as well as benefit the environment. For example, certain fish subsidies may encourage an expansion of fishing capacity beyond what the oceans can sustain in the long run; this may be aggravated by inadequate fisheries management. Where this

is the case, fewer subsidies could contribute to both reducing excessive pressure on fish stocks as well as promoting less distorted trade.

145. However, there are also risks. The fishery example also points to the importance of management structures and appropriate government regulation being in place. In many developing countries, the pace and scale of liberalization may overwhelm the capacity to develop and enforce environmental and/or occupational health regulations. In such circumstances, trade may exacerbate the consequences of poor environmental policies.

(ii) "Like products"

146. While WTO rules provide scope for Members to adopt measures aimed at achieving national environmental policies, they impose a key requirement in respect of non-discrimination. This obligation not to discriminate is closely linked to the concept of "like products" which is at the heart of many environment-related disputes. In essence this means that national environmental policies, in their application, have to treat like products similarly: products that are deemed to be "like", whether they come from different foreign suppliers or from domestic suppliers, should not be treated less favourably.

147. There are a number of specific instances in which governments may be exempted from this fundamental WTO principle. Article XX(b) and (g) are designed to allow WTO Members to adopt WTO-inconsistent policy measures if this is either necessary to protect human, animal or plant life or health, or if the measure relates to the conservation of exhaustible natural resources. The chapeau of Article XX is designed to ensure that such WTO-inconsistent measures do not result in arbitrary or unjustifiable discrimination and do not constitute a disguised restriction on international trade. In the Gasoline case (see below), a WTO dispute panel and Appellate Body ruling disallowed the 'arbitrary and unjustifiable discrimination' against foreign suppliers or producers that was involved in the US application of its environmental measure, and which violated the national treatment principle. This case is described in more detail in Box 11 below.

148. A key issue here is how health is considered when making a determination of "likeness". A recent WTO case concerning asbestos is a good illustration of this complex question.

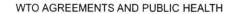

Box 11
United States - Standards for Reformulated and Conventional Gasoline (WT/DS2)

Following a 1990 amendment to the Clean Air Act, the Environmental Protection Agency (EPA) promulgated the Gasoline Rule on the composition and emissions effects of gasoline, in order to reduce air pollution in the United States and to ensure that pollution from the combustion of gasoline did not exceed 1990 levels. These rules were established to address the ozone and pollution damage experienced by large US cities, as a result, principally, of car exhaust fumes.

From 1 January 1995, the Gasoline Rule permitted only gasoline of a specified cleanliness ("reformulated gasoline") to be sold to consumers in the most polluted areas of the country. In the rest of the country, only gasoline no dirtier than that sold in the base year of 1990 ("conventional gasoline") could be sold. The Gasoline Rule applied to all US refiners, blenders and importers of gasoline.

The EPA regulation provided two different sets of baseline emissions standards. First, it required any domestic refiner which was in operation for at least six months in 1990 to establish an "individual baseline", which represented the quality of gasoline produced by that refiner in 1990.

Second, EPA established a "statutory baseline", intended to reflect average US 1990 gasoline quality. The statutory baseline was assigned to those refiners who were not in operation for at least six months in 1990, and to importers and blenders of gasoline. The statutory baseline imposed a stricter burden on foreign gasoline producers.

Venezuela and Brazil claimed that the Gasoline Rule was prejudicial to their exports to the United States and that it favoured domestic producers. Accordingly, the Gasoline Rule was inconsistent with Articles III and XXIII:1(b) of the GATT 1994, with Article 2.2 of the Agreement on Technical Barriers to Trade (TBT Agreement), and was not covered by Article XX. The United States argued that the Gasoline Rule was consistent with Article III, and, in any event, was justified under the exceptions contained in Article XX, paragraphs (b), (g) and (d), and that the Rule was also consistent with the TBT Agreement. The United States appealed the panel report but limited its appeal to the panel's interpretation of Article XX of the GATT 1994.

The panel found that imported and domestic gasoline were like products, and that since, under the baseline establishment methods, imported gasoline was effectively prevented from benefitting from sales conditions as favourable as domestic gasoline were afforded by an individual baseline tied to the producer of a product, imported gasoline was treated less favourably than domestic gasoline. The Gasoline Rule was accordingly inconsistent with Article III.

Box 11
United States - Standards for Reformulated and Conventional Gasoline (WT/DS2) (cont'd)

The panel agreed with the parties that a policy to reduce air pollution resulting from the consumption of gasoline was a policy concerning the protection of human, animal and plant life or health mentioned in Article XX(b).

However, the panel found that the baseline establishment methods were not "necessary" under Article XX(b) since there were other consistent or less inconsistent measures reasonably available to the US for the same policy objective. The panel rejected a justification of the measure under Article XX(d) as the baseline establishment methods were not an enforcement mechanism (to "secure compliance"), but were simply rules for determining the individual baselines. Finally, the panel considered that a policy to reduce the depletion of clean air was a policy to conserve a natural resource within the meaning of Article XX(g). However, the panel found that the less favourable baseline establishment methods at issue in this case were not primarily aimed at the conservation of natural resources. In light of these findings, it was not deemed necessary by the panel to determine whether the measure met the conditions set out in the chapeau of Article XX. The panel concluded that the Gasoline Rule could not be justified under Article XX(b), (d) or (g). The panel finding was reversed on appeal. The Appellate Body held that the baseline establishment rules contained in the Gasoline Rule fell within the terms of Article XX(g), but failed to meet the requirements of the chapeau of Article XX. It noted that the chapeau addressed not so much the questioned measure or its specific contents as such, but rather the manner in which that measure is applied. Accordingly, the chapeau is animated by the principle that while Members have a legal right to invoke the exceptions of Article XX, they should not be so applied as to lead to an abuse or misuse.

The Appellate Body concluded that the application of the US regulation amounted to unjustifiable discrimination and to a disguised restriction on trade because of two omissions on the part of the United States. First, the United States had not explored adequately means, including in particular cooperation with Venezuela and Brazil, of mitigating the administrative problems that led the United States to reject individual baselines for foreign refiners. Second, the United States did not count the costs for foreign refiners that would result from the imposition of statutory baselines.

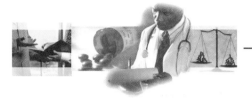

(iii) The Asbestos Case - public health takes precedence over trade

149. This case stemmed from a 1998 challenge by Canada to a complete ban by France on the import and use of chrysotile asbestos. Asbestos is the leading cause of occupational cancer and its health risks have been extensively documented. In France alone, asbestos claims the lives of about 2000 people each year and a ban on chrysotile (white) asbestos is already in place in nine of the fifteen European Union (EU) member states. France produces substitutes for asbestos, for example, polyvinyl alcohol, cellulose and glass fibres (for more detail on the case, see Box 12).

150. The Appellate Body examined whether imported asbestos fibres and domestic alternative fibres were "like products," emphasising that this question must be informed by the obligation of Members to ensure "equality of competitive conditions" between domestic products and like imports. It reiterated the classic 4 general criteria for likeness, namely (i) the physical properties of the products, (ii) their end uses, (iii) consumer tastes and habits and (iv) the tariff classification of products, emphasizing that all four criteria must be examined in all cases but that this is not a closed list and that all pertinent evidence must be taken into account. The Appellate Body found that the health risks inherent in a product may be pertinent and could influence at least two of those criteria: the physical characteristics of products and consumer tastes and habits.

151. The Asbestos case clarified the meaning of what is "necessary" to protect health under WTO rules. Once the Appellate Body had established that the ban on asbestos was designed to protect health - a vital objective - the question focused on whether any alternatives to an outright ban could be used instead. The Appellate Body ruled that France could not have reasonably been expected to employ "controlled use" practices, as Canada had contended, because "controlled use" could not be demonstrated to be effective in practice. Thus, the ban was deemed "necessary" to protect human health within the meaning of the Article XX(b) exception.

152. Just as the Thai cigarette case empowered national anti-tobacco advocates, the case inspired Brazilian environmental and occupational health advocates to push for stronger laws to protect public health. As the fifth largest producer of asbestos, Brazil filed an argument on Canada's behalf in the WTO case. However, the case strengthened arguments by civil society about the need for tougher laws on the use of asbestos. In the last two years, cities and states across Brazil - including the city of Sao Paulo, the largest city in Latin America - enacted laws banning the use of asbestos, covering about 70 per cent of the asbestos market nation-wide (International Ban Asbestos Campaign, 2000).

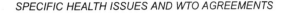

Box 12

European Communities - Measures affecting asbestos and asbestos containing products (WT/DS135)

A French Decree prohibiting the manufacture, sale, export, import and use of asbestos fibres and products containing asbestos fibres was challenged by Canada in 1998 on the grounds of less favourable treatment of imported asbestos as compared to domestic substitutes for asbestos, contrary to Article III:4 of GATT 1994. Canada also argued that banning asbestos was an unnecessarily extreme measure because the 'controlled' use of asbestos could reduce the health risks to acceptable levels. The EU argued the case on France's behalf.

In September 2000, the WTO dispute panel ruled in favour of the EU. The panel found that chrysotile asbestos and the substitute products had, inter alia, similar "end-uses", making the products alike. Thus, the French ban violated the national treatment provisions of GATT Article III.4 Nevertheless, the panel decided that France had a right to apply the ban under GATT Article XX (b) because the health risk of asbestos was substantial (Panel Report, paragraph 8.119). Canada appealed the ruling.

In March 2001, the WTO Appellate Body issued its ruling, affirming the dispute panel's ruling in favor of the EU, while clarifying several important issues:

• WTO Members have the undisputed right to determine the level of health protection they deem appropriate.

• It is appropriate to consider whether the physical characteristics influence the relative health risk of a product in evaluating its "likeness" under Article III (4) of GATT 1994. The AB agreed that evidence showed that chrysotile fibres were more toxic than the substitute products used in France and that Canada did not satisfy its burden of proving likeness.

• There is no requirement under Article XX(b) of the GATT 1994 to quantify the risk to human life or health. A risk may be evaluated either in qualitative or quantitative terms.

• Countries can base their health or environmental measures on qualified and respected scientific opinions held by only a minority of scientists: "a Member is not obliged, in setting health policy, automatically to follow what, at a given time, may constitute a majority scientific opinion" (AB report, p. 64).

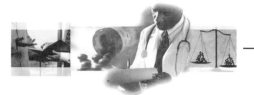

> **Box 12**
> **European Communities - Measures affecting asbestos and asbestos containing products (WT/DS135) (cont'd)**
>
> • For the Appellate Body, the determination of whether a measure which is not "indispensable" may nevertheless be "necessary" involves a process of weighing and balancing a series of factors which include the importance of the common interests or values protected by the measure, the efficacy of such measure in pursuing the policies aimed at, and the accompanying impact of the law or regulation on imports or exports.
>
> • One aspect of the "weighing and balancing process ... in the determination of whether a WTO-consistent alternative measure" is reasonably available is the extent to which the alternative measure "contributes to the realization of the end pursued". "The more vital or important [the] common interests or values" pursued, the easier it would be to accept as "necessary" measures designed to achieve those ends. In this case, the objective pursued by the measure is the preservation of human life and health through the elimination, or reduction, of the well-known, and life-threatening, health risks posed by asbestos fibres. The value pursued is both vital and important in the highest degree.
>
> • The ban was found to be "necessary" to protect health since the alternative proposed by Canada 'controlled use' of asbestos products - was not demonstrated as practical. Controlled use would pose a significant residual risk to the workers and would not, therefore, achieve the level of health protection desired by France - a halt to asbestos-induced illness and death.

(iv) Domestically prohibited goods

153. The Asbestos case recalls another issue on the WTO agenda of particular relevance to health: trade in domestically prohibited goods (DPGs). As early as 1982, concern was raised by a number of developing countries about goods being exported to them in situations where their domestic sale in the exporting countries had been either prohibited or severely restricted on health and environmental grounds.

154. At the 1982 Ministerial Meeting of GATT, it was agreed to examine the issue. Governments decided to begin notifying any goods produced and exported by them but banned for health reasons by their national authorities for sale in their domestic markets. While the notification system began to function following this Decision, Parties

tended to notify DPGs whose export had also been prohibited rather than the ones which they continued to export. The notification system was not successful, and no notifications have been received after 1990 (despite the fact that the 1982 Decision remains in force). In 1989, a Working Group on the Export of DPGs was established in GATT. The Working Group met 15 times between 1989 and 1991, when its mandate expired, but failed to resolve the issue. In the 1994 Ministerial Decision on Trade and Environment it was agreed to incorporate DPGs into the terms of reference of the Committee on Trade and the Environment (CTE). Numerous other international instruments already address the export of DPGs. This is the case with the Basel Convention on the Transboundary Movement of Hazardous Wastes as well as the PIC and POPs Conventions. These instruments principally address chemicals, pharmaceuticals, and hazardous wastes.

155. The issue of DPGs, as well as the EC-Asbestos and Thailand-Cigarette cases, illustrate some ways in which WTO agreements may influence national environmental and health policies. Other environmental policy issues relevant to trade and health include the conservation of biological diversity, environmental standards relating to the use of process and production methods and, at a more general level, the use of precaution.[35]

(v) The WTO Committee on Trade and Environment ("the CTE")

156. With the entry into force of the WTO in January 1995, the Committee on Trade and Environment was established. Its work programme builds on the work that had already taken place in GATT since 1991. The CTE has a broad-based mandate covering all areas of the multilateral trading system - goods, services and intellectual property. It has been given both analytical and prescriptive functions: to identify the relationship between trade and environmental measures in order to promote sustainable development, and to make recommendations on whether any modifications to the provisions of the multilateral trading system are required.[36] In effect, the CTE has brought environmental and sustainable development issues into the mainstream of WTO work. Perhaps a good example of this is the way the issue of fishery subsidies, which originally rose in the CTE context, was, at Doha, propelled into negotiations in the context of the Agreement on Subsidies and Countervailing Measures.

157. The CTE's first Report, which was submitted to the WTO Ministerial Conference in Singapore, notes the WTO Members' wish to approach the issue of trade and environ-

---

[35.] For a discussion of these issues and others, see Environment and Trade: A Handbook published by the UN Environment Programme and the International Institute for Sustainable Development (UNEP and IISD, 2000).

[36.] The full mandate and scope of the CTE's work programme is contained in the Ministerial Decision on Trade and Environment of 15 April 1994. This Decision establishes the Committee on Trade and Environment.

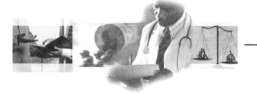

ment in a constructive manner. Trade and environment are both important areas of policy-making and they should be mutually supportive in order to promote sustainable development. At Doha, Ministers stated that they were "convinced that the aims of upholding and safeguarding an open and non-discriminatory multilateral trading system, and acting for the protection of the environment and the promotion of sustainable development *can and must* be mutually supportive" (emphasis added). Hence, the multilateral trading system has the duty to further integrate environmental considerations and enhance its contribution to the promotion of sustainable development without undermining its open, equitable and non-discriminatory character. The work of the CTE will continue to be central to achieving this objective.

(vi) Multilateral Environmental Agreements (MEAs)

158. One important aspect of the trade and environment interface is the relationship between WTO rules and multilateral environmental agreements (MEAs). As local environmental risks and trade in hazardous substances can have global and regional environmental consequences, international and regional solutions are needed. To address shared environmental problems, national governments have signed over 200 MEAs. MEAs establish shared environmental goals for those countries that ratify the agreements, and create policy guidelines for national policy development and implementation to achieve the goals. They cover issues ranging from ozone depletion to transport of hazardous waste.

159. This has been an area of particular focus in the CTE.[37] It has been clear throughout the discussions on this issue in the WTO that the preferred approach for governments to take in tackling transboundary or global environmental problems is cooperative, multilateral action under an MEA. Avoiding unilateral actions reduces the risks of arbitrary discrimination and disguised protectionism, and reflects the international community's common concern and responsibility for shared, global resources. So while MEAs are to be encouraged, the CTE has wrestled with the issue of how to address the trade provisions which several of them contain. These include trade measures agreed to among parties to MEAs, as well as measures adopted by parties to MEAs against non-parties. Allegations of conflict are concerned with trade measures contained in MEAs, given that some of the trade measures they contain violate the principle of non-discrimination. This may be the case where such measures allow for trade with some countries but not with others in like products (a violation of the most-favoured-nation principle),

37. The WTO Secretariat has prepared a note entitled "Matrix on Trade Measures Pursuant to Selected MEAs", 14 June 2001, WT/TCE/W/160/Rev.1. This matrix contains information on the provisions of 14 environmental conventions and protocols, including the recently finalized Stockholm Convention on Persistent Organic Pollutants. It is available at: www.wto.org.

or allow for discrimination between like domestic and imported products (a violation of national treatment principle).

160. In discussing the compatibility between the trade provisions contained in MEAs and GATT/WTO rules, the CTE observed that of the over 200 MEAs currently in force, just over 20 of them contain trade provisions. Therefore, the dimension of the problem should not be exaggerated. In addition, although there is potential, no disputes have thus far come to the WTO regarding the trade provisions contained in an MEA.

161. In the context of the Doha negotiations on environment, countries will be looking more closely at the relationship between existing WTO rules and specific trade obligations set out in MEAs. These negotiations will be limited in scope to the applicability of such existing WTO rules as among parties to the MEA in question. Furthermore, they are not to prejudice the WTO rights of any Member that is not a party to the MEA in question. The negotiations will also address, *inter alia*, procedures for regular information exchange between MEA Secretariats and the relevant WTO committees.

F. ACCESS TO DRUGS AND VACCINES

162. Modern medicine depends heavily on the use of drugs and vaccines to treat or prevent illness. Effective drug treatment exists for most of the leading infectious diseases, including acute respiratory infections, HIV/AIDS, malaria, diarrhoeal diseases, tuberculosis and measles. Life-saving drugs have also been developed for the leading non-communicable diseases, including ischaemic heart disease and cerebrovascular disease.

163. WHO estimates that currently one third of the world's population lacks access to essential drugs, with this figure rising to over 50% in the poorest parts of Africa and Asia (WHO, 2000b)[38]. Drugs that appear on WHO's Model List of Essential Drugs are defined as those which satisfy the health care needs of the majority of the population, should be affordable, and represent the best balance of quality, safety, efficacy and cost for a given health setting.

164. Access to essential medicines and vaccines depends on four critical elements: affordable prices, rational selection and use, sustainable financing, and reliable supply

---

[38] WHO Medicines Strategy: Framework for Action in Essential Drugs and Medicines Policy 2000-2003. Geneva: World Health Organization, 2000 (WHO/EDM/2000.1).

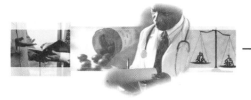

systems. Although the latter three points are equally important in order to place the problem of access to drugs in the right perspective, in health and trade discussions, the focus is usually on drug prices.

(i) Many measures will make drug prices more affordable

165. For low-income countries and poor people in particular, bringing down the cost of medicines is key to gaining access to drugs. In developing countries, 25 to 65 per cent of total health expenditures is spent on pharmaceuticals, but government health budgets are too low to purchase enough medicines and poor people often cannot afford to buy them on their own. Several measures exist for making drug prices more affordable:

(a) Price controls to restrict manufacturers' selling prices;

(b) price negotiation for high volume or pooled purchasing;

(c) reduced import duties and national or local sales taxes;

(d) distribution of price information on drug ingredients and finished doses;

(e) reduced distribution, dispensing and marketing costs;

(f) promoting competition through generic products and prompt manufacture of generic drugs upon expiration of patent terms;

(g) promoting conditions that would be conducive to differential pricing of pharmaceuticals;

(h) voluntary licensing under certain conditions for newer life-saving drugs still on patent;

(i) use of TRIPS safeguards, such as parallel imports and compulsory licensing, for patented drugs and use of exceptions to exclusive rights which permit early testing and approval of generics ("Bolar" provision).

166. A full discussion on the above aspects is beyond the scope of this document. Instead, this discussion focuses on measures likely to be affected by WTO Agreements.

(ii) Import duties and tariffs on pharmaceuticals

167. Import duties are decreasing for drugs, vaccines or other medical supplies, as global, regional and bilateral agreements to reduce tariffs come into effect. Average tariffs on final pharmaceutical products are generally low or moderate in the developing

world, with the exception of only a few countries, such as India and Tunisia, where they are 30 and 20.6 per cent respectively. For active ingredients that go into the manufacture of pharmaceuticals, six developing countries have average tariffs in the range of 20 to 30 per cent (Burkina Faso, Pakistan, Tanzania, India, Kenya and Tunisia).[39]
Some developing countries allow a limited number of essential drugs to enter duty free. And a few, mostly developed WTO Members have committed themselves in their WTO tariff schedules to grant duty-free access for pharmaceutical products.[40] There may be some potential for price reductions on pharmaceuticals through lower import duties.

168. There appears to be some scope for further lowering of import tariffs on other health-related products. Studies on barriers to trade in anti-malaria supplies showed that import tariffs on mosquito nets and insecticides in sub-Saharan African countries added from 20 to 40 per cent to their price in Sub-Saharan Africa (PATH/Canada, 1998 and Simon et al, 2001)[41]. Uganda's decision to eliminate import duties on anti-malaria bed nets, and Tanzania's lowering of the taxes, represent important efforts to make such preventive health measures more affordable (see Box 13).

Box 13
Uganda ends "malaria taxes"

In its June 2000 budget, Uganda eliminated taxes and import tariffs on mosquito nets and insecticides used to fight malaria. Uganda was the first country to act on this pledge made by African Heads of State at the African Malaria Summit in April 2000. Tanzania was the first African country to take action on the 'malaria tax; in 1999, it reduced the total of taxes and tariff duty to 5 per cent, making mosquito nets more affordable, averaging US$3.50.

Prices for nets vary widely across Africa, with prices reported to be as high as US$45 in Swaziland and US$30 in Sudan - putting them out of reach of most Africans. Utilization rates also vary widely, but may be in the order of 10-30 per cent overall, and cost is a major constraint. Eliminating tariffs could increase utilization. Most tax and tariff authorities continue to view insecticide-treated nets as textiles, instead of classifying them as pharmaceutical materials with the potential to save lives.

---

[39]. Internal study by the WTO and UNCTAD Secretariats (2000, unpublished).

[40]. This arrangement was drawn up during the Uruguay Round and subsequently expanded in coverage. The countries concerned are: Canada, the Czech Republic, the European Communities, Japan, Macau, Norway, the Slovak Republic, Switzerland and the United States.

[41]. Restricted Trade? Barriers to Trade in Mosquito Nets and Insecticides in sub-Saharan African. Ottawa: Programme for Appropriate Technology in Health (PATH) Canada, 1998.
Simon, J., Larson, B., Rosen, S. and Zusman, A. et al. Reducing Tariffs and Taxes on Insecticide Treated Bednets. Background Paper for Africa Malaria Day, 2001.

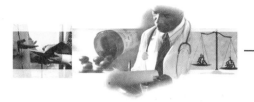

(iii) Impact of patent protection and the TRIPS Agreement on the availability of drugs

169. An assessment of the impact of patent protection on access to drugs and vaccines needs to address the balance that is found in the patent regime between:

- the effect of patent protection in promoting the invention, development and marketing of new drugs, by providing incentives for research and development;
- the effect of patent protection in limiting access to existing drugs and vaccines.

170. An analysis of the extent to which these effects can be attributed to the TRIPS Agreement depends on assumptions about what would have happened in the absence of the Agreement. The TRIPS Agreement resulted from a long and complex negotiation in which countries brought their different interests and perspectives to bear. As is made clear in Section II of this paper, it represents an effort to find a balance between the sometimes conflicting considerations referred to in the previous paragraph. On the one hand, it obliges all WTO Member countries to provide protection for product and process patents, including in the areas of pharmaceuticals and vaccines, for a minimum of 20 years from filing. On the other hand, it enshrines in international public law certain rights that all countries have to implement their patent and other intellectual property regimes in a way which takes into account public health and other public policy objectives. The provisions on compulsory licensing and parallel imports are those most frequently referred to in this connection. What would have been the outcome in the absence of agreed multilateral rules and if the resolution of international differences in this area had been left to bilateral processes is impossible to know, although the provisions of bilateral agreements give some indicators.

171. While the TRIPS Agreement may have some effects in countries which already provided product patent protection for pharmaceuticals, for example by virtue of the lengthening of the term of patent protection, the most marked effects will be in those countries that are obliged by their TRIPS obligations to introduce such protection. To assess the impact of the TRIPS Agreement in these countries, it is necessary to examine, *inter alia*, the following factors:

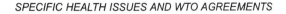

- the timing of the impact, given the TRIPS transition arrangements;
- the proportion of drugs on the market that will be covered by patent protection, and the importance of these for basic health care; and
- the effect of patent protection on prices, taking into account the safeguards permitted under the TRIPS Agreement.

(iv) Patent protection provides incentives for R&D into new drugs

172. While the importance of patent protection is providing incentives for R&D into pharmaceuticals is widely accepted (see Box 14), there is a debate about the extent to which patent protection for pharmaceuticals in developing countries adds to these incentives. The questions are, first, to what extent does a world-wide requirement to protect pharmaceuticals inventions at the level of TRIPS standards enhance the overall level of incentives for R&D into diseases in general and, secondly, to what extent will such a requirement affect incentives in the case of diseases which predominantly afflict people in developing countries. While there have been some studies of the effect of the introduction of pharmaceutical patent protection on the level of local R&D in the countries that have introduced it,[42] there does not appear to have been a study which has specifically addressed this overall aspect. However, one expert in this area has observed that extension of product patent protection as a result of TRIPS could result in a rise in demand of as much as 25 per cent of global spending on patented drugs, even without taking into account the case of China (Lanjouw, 1997).[43] Nonetheless, widespread concern has also been expressed that, left to itself, the patent system, even after TRIPS implementation, will not lead to sufficient incentives for R&D into the diseases prevalent amongst the poor in developing countries, such as malaria. This has led to widespread consideration of supplementary action at the international level, both in terms of so-called "push" mechanisms, involving financial contributions towards R&D, and so-called "pull" mechanisms, aimed at ensuring the existence of an attractive level of demand in the event that successful drugs or vaccines are generated. Examples of internationally sponsored public/private partnerships to address these problems are the Medicines for Malaria Venture (MMV) and the International AIDS Vaccine Initiative (IAVI).

---

42. These studies include: Nogues, 1990 (Argentina); Kawaura and LaCroix, 1995 (Korea); Scherer and Weisburst, 1995 (Italy); LaCroix and Kawaura, 1996 (Japan); Lanjouw, 1997 (India); Maskus, 1997 (Lebanon); Korenko, 1999 (Italy); Lanjouw and Cockburn, 2000 (India). The results vary from study to study and no general picture seems to emerge.

43. Lanjouw, J.O. The Introduction of Product Patents in India: "Heartless Exploitation of the Poor and Suffering"?, Growth Center Discussion Paper, Yale University, and NBER Working Paper no. 6366, 1997.

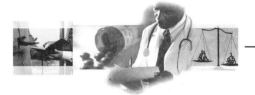

Box 14
Effect of the patent system in promoting the invention, development and marketing of new drugs

A key function of the patent system is to provide incentives for research and development into new inventions, by giving inventors exclusive rights over their inventions for a limited period of time. Several studies try to answer the questions of whether, in general, strong intellectual property protection stimulates investment in R&D and, in particular, pharmaceutical patent protection encourages the development of new drugs.

This is important because it is possible that innovation and technological development in the private sector may possibly be spurred by factors other than patents, such as commercial rivalry, market conditions and technical barriers to imitation. Indeed, studies based on firm-level surveys (Mansfield, 1986; Levin et al, 1987) showed that in most industries these other factors are the most important instruments in capturing the returns from R&D investments. However, these studies found that, in the pharmaceuticals and chemicals sectors, patents were seen as the most important factor for R&D decisions and the development of new products. In a recent and more extensive study (Cohen et al, 2000), these findings were broadly reaffirmed. Overall, for all US industry groups studied, lead time, trade secrets and complementary manufacturing, sales and service efforts were seen as more important than patents in appropriating the fruits of innovation. But again, this study confirmed that it was the pharmaceutical sector, with the medical equipment sector, that gave the highest score to patent protection. This study suggests that secrecy, lead time and complementary manufacturing capability are also of high importance in the pharmaceutical industry.

Scherer (2000) suggests that there could be three probable reasons for the special importance of patents to pharmaceutical innovation. First, patents for new pharmaceuticals, unlike for new products in many other areas of industry, give effective protection since patent claims can be defined more precisely for chemical molecules, thus making it relatively easier to prove infringement. Second, pharmaceutical R&D costs are particularly high and so the legal protection offered by patents is especially important to secure the commercial benefits.[44]

Third, in the absence of protection, imitation costs would be low given that knowledge created by originator firms in the therapeutic value and safety and efficacy of the molecule can be used by others with very low costs.

44. *For instance, studies have shown that the US pharmaceutical industry devoted the largest fraction of its revenue to R&D from among 230 industries: this proportion has been increasing over time to reach a current level of around 20 percent (Scherer, 2000, 1302).*

Box 14
Effect of the patent system in promoting the invention, development and marketing of new drugs (cont'd)

A further factor which appears to differentiate the pharmaceutical industry from many other industries is the relatively long life-span of pharmaceutical inventions and the corresponding lower significance of lead time as a factor for appropriating benefits.[45]

With regard to the average cost of producing a new, innovative drug, industry circles place the figure at around US$ 500 million (IFPMA, 1998, 9). A recent study published by an NGO (Public Citizen, 2001) claims that it could be closer to US$ 100 million or less, even taking account of industry data. Both claims base their estimates on data provided in an earlier study (DiMasi et al, 1991), the author of which placed the average cost of developing a new drug at US$ 231 million in 1987. This study has been updated by the same author and the cost (in 2000) is placed at c.$800 million per new drug. The increase has been attributed to increased costs of drug development, particularly in the clinical testing period.[46] A further aspect of the innovative pharmaceutical industry that is often discussed in relation to the degree of incentive required for R&D is the element of risk. Industry generally claims that the industry is particularly risky, relying on a relatively small number of so-called "blockbuster products" for the bulk of profits and with a very large number of drugs that fail to break even. There are studies which support this view (Scherer, 2000; Grabowski and Vernon, 1990, 1994). On the other hand, the Public Citizen study referred to above concludes that pharmaceutical R&D does not appear to be particularly risky because that most new drugs are "me-too" drugs (i.e. they constitute close substitutes for successful drugs) and that publicly funded research accounts for the initial R&D costs of many important drugs.

Given that, other things being equal, patents constitute a means by which companies can charge higher prices, a vital issue is whether there is a real link between increased profitability and increased R&D in the pharmaceutical industry. Until recently there has not been a serious study examining this relationship. However, a recent study (Scherer, 2001) has shown a strong link and concludes that the evidence shows that, as profit opportunities expand, firms will compete to exploit them by increasing R&D investments. This study, which was based on a time-series analysis of data for the US pharmaceutical industry for more than 30 years on R&D investment and industry profits, showed a striking similarly of both data series in deviations from the time trend.

[45] *This is indicated, for example, by studies which show the relatively high proportion of pharmaceutical patents for which renewal fees are paid and which remain valid for their full term compared to other product areas.*
[46] *See http://www.tufts.edu/med/csdd/Nov30CostStudyPressRelease.html*

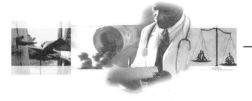

(v) Concern that TRIPS could lead to higher prices for some drugs

173. International conventions before TRIPS did not specify most of the minimum standards for patents. Over 40 countries provided no product patent protection for pharmaceuticals prior to the launching of the negotiation of the TRIPS Agreement and some 20 WTO Members still did not do so by the time of the conclusion of the TRIPS negotiations. A few of these countries did not provide process protection in this area as well. The duration of patents was less than 20 years in many countries. One effect of patent protection is that it gives the patent owner the right to prevent the competition from using the information to produce the same products and the possibility to set prices higher than they could otherwise. For this reason, the price of patented drugs is often much higher than the price that would prevail if generic competition were allowed. Such differences lie behind the concern that TRIPS could result in substantial increases in the price of drugs once countries implement its rules.

174. Simple price comparisons, however, using current exchange rates, are often made of the prices of new, patented medicines in countries with pharmaceutical patent protection (typically the United States) and in those without (typically India) to conclude that patents lead to higher prices.[47] However, such price comparisons are problematic as they do not isolate the effect of patents from those of other demand and supply factors such as purchasing power and cost of production. It is possible that there are also major price differences in the price of non-patented items of consumption, including medicines. Moreover, there is evidence that the absence of patent protection and the presence of a number of generic producers do not always mean lower priced drugs, as in the case of Argentina for HIV/AIDS drugs indicators.[48]

175. However, macro-level studies comparing drug prices across countries find that those with the most stringent patent protection laws have higher pharmaceutical prices on average than those with less stringent patent laws (Scherer, 1993).[49] Economic modelling studies have estimated mean price increases for new pharmaceutical products, using assumptions that give the highest impact, to be over 200 per cent after the intro-

---

47. For example, fluconazole, a drug used to treat deadly fungal infections related to HIV/AIDS, costs around $10 a pill wholesale in the US where the branded version of the drugs is under patent and the manufacturer has exclusive rights. It has sold for just 25 cents a tablet in India, where a local manufacturer produces a copy because India's current patent law does not cover product patents until 2005 (The Lancet, Access to fluconazole in less developed countries, Volume 356, Number 9247, 16 December 2000).

48. For further details see the background paper prepared by the WTO consultant for the WHO-WTO Secretariat workshop on differential pricing and financing of essential drugs held in Norway in April 2001 and available on the WTO web site.

49. Scherer, F.M. Pricing, profits, and technological progress in the pharmaceutical Industry. The Journal of Economic Perspectives, 1993, 7: 97-115.

duction of product patents (Challu,1991; Fink, 2000; Watal, 2000).[50] Such models are highly sensitive to the methodologies used and the assumptions made. Changing the assumptions, the average price effect has been estimated as less than 30 per cent (Watal, 2000). It should be emphasized, however, that these studies do not take into account the flexibility available in the TRIPS Agreement, for example compulsory licensing, government use and parallel importation, nor the possible use of price or similar controls, which is not regulated by the TRIPS Agreement. A detailed study of the Indian market concluded that "the combination of ... low purchasing power, price control or reserve powers under pricing freedom and therapeutic competition ... enable one to predict with some confidence that there will be no general 'price explosion' in India either with or without patent protection" (Redwood, 1994).[51]

176. There are few empirical studies for specific countries showing the actual effects of their introducing patents for pharmaceuticals. This is because the price of drugs depends on many factors - supply and demand; prescribing and consumption patterns; manufacturing costs; competitive conditions in the markets; taxes, exchange rates, and royalty payments for patented drugs; wholesale and retail mark-ups; degree of price elasticity for different drugs; and especially, government or private health plan coverage and payment policies. Thus, distinguishing the price effects attributable to newly introduced patent protection involves methodological difficulties (Scherer and Watal, draft 2001)[52]. A recent study from Thailand that tackled some of these problems found no significant price changes due to the introduction of product patent protection (Supakankunti, et al., 2001).[53]

177. Owing to the inconclusive nature of the studies conducted to date, and because of the effect that potentially significant price increases could have on access to drugs in poor countries, WHO is currently monitoring and evaluating the effects of TRIPS on the prices of medicines. It is also monitoring the TRIPS impact on other important issues such as transfer of technology, levels of research and development for drugs for neglected diseases, and the evolution of generic drug markets.

---

[50] Challu, P.M. The consequences of pharmaceutical product patenting. World Competition, 1991, 15(2): 65-126

Fink, C. "How Stronger Patent Protection in India Might Affect the Behavior of Transnational Pharmaceutical Industries". World Bank, May 2000.

Watal J. Pharmaceutical patents, prices and welfare losses: policy options for India under the WTO TRIPS Agreement. World Economy, 2000, 23: 733-752.

[51] Redwood, H. New horizons in India: The consequences of pharmaceutical patent protection, Oldwicks Press, Suffolk, 1994

[52] Scherer, F.M., Watal J. Post - TRIPS options for access to patented medicines in developing countries. Commission on Macroeconomics and Health. 2001,Working Group 4, Paper 1.

[53] Supakankunti S. et al., Impact of the World Trade Organization TRIPS Agreement on the pharmaceutical industry in Thailand, Bulletin of the World Health Organization, 2001, Volume 79, Number 5: 461-470.

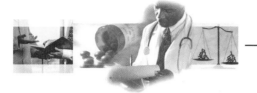

178. While some new drugs may be more expensive in some countries as a result of more widespread patent protection, it is important to keep the extent of the problem in perspective. The vast majority of the 300 or so drugs on WHO's Model List of Essential Drugs are not under patent protection in any country. The need to implement patent protection according to TRIPS standards will not, in general, affect the price of drugs now on the WHO model list. The cost and affordability of drugs have been among the criteria for inclusion in the WHO model list, so the limited number of patented drugs on the model list does not necessarily reflect the actual need for key patent-protected life-saving drugs by people in developing countries. But the fact that billions of people lack access to essential drugs, most of which are not protected by patents, underscores the other problems contributing to inadequate access - poorly developed supply and distribution systems, lack of financing, lack of generic drug production or import capacity, and affordability of even generic drugs for people in poorer countries.

179. In addition, most developing countries already provided product patent protection for pharmaceuticals prior to the entry into force of the TRIPS Agreement and, of those that did not, some have introduced it prior to the end of the transition period to which they are entitled under the TRIPS Agreement (2005 for developing countries and 2016 for least-developed countries [54]). Furthermore, developing countries not already providing patent protection to pharmaceutical products are only required to implement such protection for drugs or vaccines that were new for patentability purposes after the end of 1994. TRIPS rules are therefore, "less of an issue for the vast share of existing [off-patent] drugs than it is for new and future essential drugs patented after 1995." (Loewenson, 2000).[55] The impact of the TRIPS rules in these countries has not been or will not be immediate, as the new products covered by the patents take time to be developed and obtain marketing approval. As a result, the impact of these TRIPS rules in those developing countries began gradually after 2000, with full impact only by 2015. Nor are patent protection requirements a significant deterrent to the utilization of most vaccines currently on the market in developing countries, although it should be noted that the structure of the vaccine market differs considerably from that of the pharmaceutical market in the context of the TRIPS Agreement (see Box 15). Yet, some of the most effective new drugs to combat HIV/AIDS, malaria and tuberculosis - diseases that inflict enormous human and economic loss - were invented after 1995[56] and as such will be entitled to patent protection in more developing countries.

[54.] See Articles 65.2, 65.4 and 66.1, and the Doha Declaration on the TRIPS Agreement and public health.

[55.] Loewenson, R. Essential Drugs in Southern Africa Need Protection from Public Health Safeguards under TRIPS, BRIDGES 4:7 September 2000: 18-23

[56.] The effective period of patent protection for pharmaceuticals that use new chemical entities is very much shorter than the nominal 20-year period, especially in developing countries, because of the time taken to obtain marketing approval from the public health authorities.

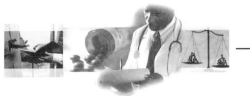

Box 15
What is the difference between vaccines and other pharmaceuticals in the context of TRIPS?

Vaccines have the following special characteristics:

1. There are relatively few vaccine manufacturers. These manufacturers work closely with the public sector to ensure a reliable supply of essential vaccines, and to facilitate technology transfer through partnerships and joint ventures.

2. Vaccines are a heat-sensitive biological product. Since they are administered to healthy children, often by injection, the safety and quality requirements for vaccines are very high. Therefore, their procurement and distribution are strictly controlled. In addition, essential vaccines are usually provided free of charge to consumers, greatly reducing the likelihood of leakage, resale, and piracy.

3. A significant amount of "know how" is needed in order to produce a vaccine. This know how is not communicated through process or product patents. For this reason, compulsory licensing is unlikely to be an effective means of transferring vaccine production capacity.

Does patent protection restrict access to essential vaccines? Until recently there has been about a 15 year lag between the introduction of a new vaccine in the developed world, and its uptake in developing countries. Clearly, the higher prices of relatively new vaccines are one of the barriers to their adoption, and royalties do contribute to the cost of vaccine production. However, WHO experts note that utilization is no greater for off-patent vaccines than for patented vaccines against the same antigen, even where they are equally effective. This has been shown for hepatitis B and acellular pertussis. Furthermore, the contribution of royalties to selling price is generally in the range of zero to six per cent. In general, patent protection does not appear to be a major barrier to current vaccine uptake and utilization in developing countries.

(vi) However, the TRIPS Agreement contains public health safeguards

180. The TRIPS Agreement affords discretion to WTO Members in how its obligations are implemented, as long as national laws conform to the minimum standards under the Agreement. In discussions leading up to the TRIPS Agreement, it was argued that unqualified IPR rights are not necessarily appropriate for countries struggling to meet health and development needs. Developing and other countries can therefore use the flexibility of TRIPS provisions and its safeguards to protect public health. These are dis-

cussed in more detail in section II above of this paper, but three of the most important are compulsory licensing, parallel imports and measures to enable the early introduction of generics. There are also important measures that can be taken outside the field of intellectual property.

Making generic drugs available upon patent expiration

181. To keep drug prices affordable, many countries promote the production or importation of generic versions of essential medicines. Until a recent WTO dispute panel ruling involving Canada and the EU (see Box 16), however, it was unclear whether the TRIPS Agreement allowed governments to permit generic drug manufacturers to undertake and complete the task of obtaining regulatory approval from the public health authorities for their generic version before the expiry of the patent term. The dispute panel ruled that TRIPS allows generic drug manufacturers, without the permission of the patent holder, to produce and/or import and use quantities necessary to conduct bioequivalency and other tests and to submit samples needed to obtain regulatory approval before the expiry of a patent. This allows generic drugs to be placed on the market more quickly than if this work had to wait until the patent actually expired. As noted in Chapter 2, this policy is sometimes referred to as the "Bolar Exception", after a similar provision in US patent law. The dispute panel clarified, however, that TRIPS does not permit "stock-piling" or large-scale commercial production of the generic drug before the patent expires.

Box 16
WTO Dispute: Canada - Patent protection of pharmaceutical products, complaint by the European Communities (WT/DS114/1)

In late 1997, the European Community contended that Canada's laws did not provide adequate protection of patented pharmaceutical inventions by allowing domestic generic pharmaceutical makers to conduct tests and carry out other preparations for producing a drug before a patent expired, without the patent holders approval, and to stockpile generic drugs six months before a drug's patent expires - alleged violations of TRIPS Article 27.1, 28.1 and 33.

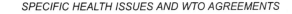

Box 16
WTO Dispute: Canada - Patent protection of pharmaceutical products, complaint by the European Communities (WT/DS114/1) (cont'd)

Canada countered that its laws were valid exceptions under Article 30, which allows "limited exceptions to the exclusive rights conferred by a patent."

In March 2000, the dispute panel validated the Canadian law allowing generic drug makers to test patented drugs or undertake other actions necessary for the purposes of seeking marketing approval for their generic versions or file for licences prior to the patent's expiration. But it found that stockpiling of generic products was not permitted under TRIPS Article 28. According to the Panel ruling, the key issue was whether stockpiling with no restrictions on amount could constitute a "limited" exception to patent owner's rights. "With no limitations at all upon the quantity of production, the stockpiling exception removes that protection entirely during the last six months of the patent term, without regard to what other, subsequent, consequences it might have. By this effect alone, the stockpiling exception can be said to abrogate such rights entirely during the time it is in effect." (WT/DS114/R, para. 7.33). Thus, manufacturers must wait until patent expiry before starting commercial production. According to an article at the time, "Generic drug manufactures note that the ruling would result in only modest production delays for generic drugs, but goes a long way to protect consumer interests by cutting time-to-market for generic drugs by as much as two to three years" ("DSB Rules On Generic Drugs", Bridges, 8 February 2000, International Centre for Trade and Sustainable Development, Geneva).

Compulsory licensing (and government use)

182. Compulsory licensing enables a competent government authority to license the use of an invention to a third party or government agency without the consent of the patent-holder. National laws in most developed and developing countries provide for the granting of compulsory licenses, which is an important component of any comprehensive national patent regime. In some countries, compulsory licenses have been used more particularly in the pharmaceutical sector to stimulate price-lowering competition and to ensure, *inter alia*, availability of needed medicines.

183. Compulsory licensing is one way in which TRIPS attempts to strike a balance between promoting access to existing drugs and promoting research and development into new drugs. It is explicitly allowed by the TRIPS Agreement subject to certain con-

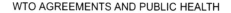
ditions set out in Article 31 (see Section 2). The Doha Declaration on the TRIPS Agreement and Public Health clarifies some of these provisions, while maintaining Members' commitments in the TRIPS Agreement. It makes it clear that each Member is free to determine the grounds upon which compulsory licences may be granted. This, for example, is a useful corrective to the views often expressed in some quarters implying that some form of emergency is a pre-condition for compulsory licensing. The TRIPS Agreement does refer to national emergencies or other circumstances of extreme urgency in connection with compulsory licensing, but only to indicate that in these circumstances the usual condition that an effort must first be made to seek a voluntary licence does not apply. The Declaration makes it clear that each Member has the right to determine what constitutes a national emergency or other circumstances of extreme urgency and that public health crises, including those relating to HIV/AIDS, tuberculosis, malaria and other epidemics, can represent such circumstances.

184. In the work on the Declaration the issue arose of the ability of countries with limited manufacturing capacities to make effective use of compulsory licensing. It is not in dispute that Members can issue compulsory licences for importation as well as for domestic production. However, concern has been expressed as to whether sources of supply from generic producers in other countries to meet such demand will be available, particularly in the light of the provision of Article 31(f) of the TRIPS Agreement which states that any compulsory licences granted to generic producers in those other countries shall be "predominantly for the supply of the domestic market of the Member" granting the compulsory licence. This concern may become greater as countries with important generic industries, such as India, come under an obligation to provide patent protection for pharmaceutical products as from 2005. In this regard, the Declaration recognizes the problem and instructs the Council for TRIPS to find an expeditious solution and submit a report before the end of 2002.

Parallel imports

185. Parallel imports enable a country to take advantage of products which the right holder has put on the market in another country at a lower price. As mentioned in Section 2, in view of Article 6, TRIPs, if a country allows parallel imports, this cannot be raised as a dispute in the WTO unless fundamental principles of non-discrimination are involved. There has been much debate about what exactly this means in regard to a Member's freedom to choose its own regime for exhaustion and parallel imports. The

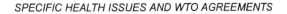

Doha Declaration on the TRIPS Agreement and Public Health makes it clear that the effect of the provisions in the TRIPS Agreement on exhaustion is to leave each Member free to establish its own regime without challenge - subject to the general TRIPS provisions prohibiting discrimination on the basis of the nationality of persons.

Measures outside the field of intellectual property

186. The scope afforded in the TRIPS Agreement for domestic regulation and a government's health policy in general is an important part of the "balance" in the Agreement. Governments have available a range of public policy measures outside the field of intellectual property to address issues of access to and prices of drugs. For example, many countries use price or reimbursement controls. Article 8 of the TRIPS Agreement makes it clear that WTO Members may, in formulating or amending their rules and regulations, adopt measures necessary to protect public health and nutrition, provided that such measures are consistent with the provisions of the Agreement.

187. Where patent protection confers pricing power for drugs of vital public health or life-saving importance, differential pricing is one way of ensuring that prices in poor developing countries are as low as possible while higher prices in rich countries continue to provide incentives for R&D. Also called "tiered" or "equity" pricing, differential pricing involves charging lower prices in poorer countries and thus spreading the burden of providing incentives for research and development more equitably. The TRIPS Agreement does not stand in the way of such arrangements.

188. The WHO and WTO Secretariats jointly organized a workshop for interested parties in April 2001 in Høsbjør, Norway to examine the legal, institutional and political environment that would favour widespread use of differential pricing and how the practice could be used and promoted to improve poor countries' access to essential drugs.[57] The meeting reviewed several options for implementing differential pricing, including: bilateral negotiation of price discounts between companies and governments; use of bulk purchasing power; and voluntary or compulsory licensing arrangements. Participants emphasized that global mechanisms or international cooperation would be needed to support some of these options. It was also pointed out that the TRIPS Agreement does not affect decisions to set different prices for drugs, nor would differential pricing require countries to forego any flexibility they have under the TRIPS Agreement. But the workshop left unanswered some key questions. How can the most

---

57. The report of this workshop is available on the WTO website (www.wto.org).

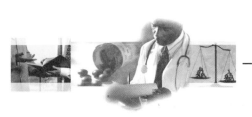
favourable price, sometimes referred to as marginal cost or not-for-profit price, be determined? What types of incentives would be most effective for encouraging differential pricing? How, in political terms can pricing in developed countries be insulated from differential pricing in poor countries, including in regard to the use of reference pricing systems? What are the best ways of securing effective separation of markets and preventing trade diversion, while taking into account international trade rules? How should middle-income developing countries and well-to-do populations in poor countries be treated under differential pricing?

189. An example of a differential pricing strategy in action is the voluntary price-cuts by several big drug companies announced in the last few years, in which the price of certain drugs for the treatment of HIV and AIDS was reduced by 90 per cent or more. However, even at such reduced prices, the cost may still be prohibitive for the poorest countries.

190. One way of addressing this problem is the donation of drugs by pharmaceutical companies, as an important contribution to making essential drugs affordable to the poorest countries. Even so, donations are not considered to be a long-term solution to the affordability problem because of their time-limited nature. According to the WHO background paper for the WHO-WTO meeting on differential pricing, donation programmes, "can make major contributions to better global public health, particularly when directed at time-limited needs such as disease eradication. At the same time, for many of the most common problems responsible for high disease burdens, donated drugs are unlikely to be a sustainable solution to meeting long-term country needs." The prospects of such contributions providing a sustainable solution may be enhanced where they are accompanied by measures by developed country governments, such as tax incentives.

191. What is clear, however, is that low prices and even donations cannot substitute for the need for the international community to provide greater financial support for health care in the poorest countries, both for the reinforcement of the local health care system and for the purchase of drugs, vaccines and goods necessary for other forms of treatment or preventive care. One such initiative is the Global Fund proposed by UN Secretary-General Kofi Annan dedicated to the battle against HIV/AIDS and other infectious diseases.

(vii) The right to use compulsory licensing under the TRIPS Agreement, and the issue of parallel imports: experiences of some countries

192. A good deal of concern has recently been expressed about whether the right of countries to use the public health safeguards provided for in the TRIPS Agreement is sufficiently recognized and accepted. Given that developing countries have only recently come under an obligation to comply with TRIPS norms, the evidence on difficulties in using TRIPS safeguards is limited. However, the concern has been sufficiently widespread for the WTO Council for TRIPS to initiate a work programme aimed at clarifying the flexibility available in the TRIPS Agreement, so as to give greater legal certainty and security in its use.

193. Part of this concern has resulted from the fact that, at the end of the Uruguay Round, at least one WTO Member, the United States, did not accept that the standards of protection of intellectual property provided for in the TRIPS Agreement were necessarily adequate and decided that it would continue to seek higher standards of protection through other means, including its procedures under the Special Section 301 of its Trade Act. However, in May 2000, the US Government issued an executive order stating its commitment to refrain from actions intended to seek the revocation or revision of intellectual property laws applying to HIV/AIDS-related drugs or technologies, provided that they were TRIPS-consistent (see Box 17). The executive order extended to measures being introduced by sub-Saharan African countries to address the HIV/AIDS endemic. In February 2001, the Bush administration reaffirmed the commitment of the United States to a flexible approach on health and intellectual property and the United States has since informed WTO Members that, as the United States takes steps to address major health crises, such as the HIV/AIDS crisis in sub-Saharan Africa and elsewhere, it would raise no objection if Members availed themselves of the flexibility afforded by the TRIPS Agreement.[58]

---

58. US statement on intellectual property and access to medicines at the 20 June 2001 TRIPS Council meeting, available at http://www.ustr.gov/sectors/speech01.pdf.

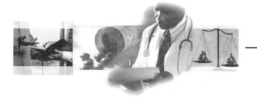

Box 17

US White House Executive Order 13155, May 20, 2000 - Access To HIV/AIDS pharmaceuticals and medical technologies

"In administering sections 301-310 of the Trade Act of 1974, the United States shall not seek, through negotiation or otherwise, the revocation or revision of any intellectual property law or policy of a beneficiary sub-Saharan African country, as determined by the President, that regulates HIV/AIDS pharmaceuticals or medical technologies if the law or policy of the country: (1) promotes access to HIV/AIDS pharmaceuticals or medical technologies for affected populations in that country; and (2) provides adequate and effective intellectual property protection consistent with the Agreement on Trade-Related Aspects of Intellectual Property Rights (TRIPS Agreement) referred to in section 101(d)(15) of the Uruguay Round Agreements Act (19 U.S.C. 3511(d)(15))."

---

194. Two cases relevant to the use of the flexibility in the TRIPS Agreement that have arisen in the WTO are often referred to. One is the dispute between Canada and the European Communities in which the WTO panel endorsed the compatibility of the "regulatory" or so-called "Bolar" exception with the TRIPS Agreement, but found against the stock-piling provision in the Canadian law (see para. 59 above for further details).

195. The other was a complaint brought under the WTO dispute settlement system in May 2000 by the United States against a provision of the Brazilian industrial property law of 1996. The provision in question had not been used and therefore the dispute was about the consistency of the Brazilian legal framework for the grant of compulsory licences with the provisions of the TRIPS Agreement. In its request for establishment of a panel, the United States alleged that Article 68 of Brazil's 1996 industrial property law, imposes a "local working" requirement which stipulates that a patent shall be subject to compulsory licensing if the subject matter of the patent is not "worked" in the territory of Brazil. Specifically, the United States challenged the provision whereby it claimed that a compulsory license shall be granted on a patent if the patented product is not manufactured in Brazil or if the patented process is not used in Brazil. In addition, according to the United States, if a patent owner chooses to exploit the patent through importation rather than "local working," then Article 68 would allow others to import either the patented product or the product obtained from the patented process. The United States argued that Article 68 of Brazil's 1996 industrial property law discrimi-

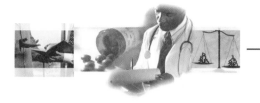

nates against US owners of Brazilian patents whose products are imported into, but not locally produced in, Brazil. Article 68 was also said to curtail the exclusive rights conferred on these owners by their patents. For the United States such legislation was part of an industrial policy.

196. Brazil contested the industrial policy nature of its challenged provision. It argued on the contrary that its legislation was compatible with TRIPS and referred to the US requirements as being contrary to and above the TRIPS standards. For Brazil, its legislation was not discriminatory and in fact it contained provisions parallel to those of Sections 204 and 209 of the US Patent Code, in particular with regard to the local working requirements. According to Brazil, under Section 204 "Preference for the United States Industry", the US Patent Code required that small business firms and universities that receive federal funding "manufacture substantially" their inventions in the United States. For Brazil, Section 209 of the same Code also established a local working requirement for federally owned patents. Brazil indeed requested consultations regarding the TRIPS compatibility of the said US legislation.[59] Since the dispute was settled before parties exchanged any formal written submission,[60] it is difficult to know with accuracy all the arguments that were put forward during the bilateral consultations or that could have been raised by the parties.

197. In June 2001, Brazil and the United States settled their WTO dispute.[61] The United States withdrew its WTO complaint against Brazil, while Brazil agreed that if it deemed it necessary to apply Article 68 to issue a compulsory license on patents held by US companies, it would hold prior bilateral talks with the US. The US indicated that it expected that Brazil would not proceed with its challenge of US legislation on the ground that it requires local working. The parties explicitly considered the agreement, "an important step towards greater cooperation between the two countries regarding our shared goals of fighting AIDS and protecting intellectual property rights." It should also be noted that Brazil has successfully used, on at least two occasions, the threat of compulsory licensing to secure more favourable terms in its negotiations for the supply of HIV/AIDS drugs with major pharmaceutical companies.

198. Another case which has attracted much attention is the challenge in the South African courts by 39 companies contending that the South African Medicines and Related Substances Control Amendment Act of 1997 was inconsistent with the South African

---

[59.] See document WT/DS 224/1.

[60.] The United States requested the establishment of a Panel (Brazil - Measures Affecting Patent Protection, complaint by the United States (WT/DS199/3)) in January 2001. A panel was established in February 2001 and Cuba, the Dominican Republic, Honduras, India and Japan reserved their third party rights.

[61.] On 5 July 2001, the parties to the dispute notified to the DSB a mutually satisfactory solution on the matter (WT/DS199/4).

Constitution. The background of this domestic dispute is the following. In 1997 the Parliament of South Africa adopted the Medicines and Related Substances Control Amendment Act (the "Medicines Amendment Act") to assist in implementation of its 1996 National Drug Policy. That Policy was designed "to ensure an adequate and reliable supply of safe, cost-effective drugs of acceptable quality to all citizens of South Africa and rational use of drugs by prescribers, dispensers and consumers" (National Drug Policy for South Africa, Department of Health, January 1996). The Medicines Amendment Act included several key components, among them provisions on generic substitution of prescription drugs, rationalization of pricing and reform of the Medicines Control Council. The Medicines Amendment Act empowered the Minister of Health to authorize and prescribe conditions for the parallel importation of drugs under patent in South Africa.

199. Prior to the provisions of the Medicines Amendment Act taking effect, 39 pharmaceutical companies sued the South African Government in order to block its implementation. The companies alleged that the Act was inconsistent with the newly adopted Constitution of South Africa in that it authorized the Minister to abrogate the rights of patent holders and violated the terms of the TRIPS Agreement. The Government argued that its legislation was entirely consistent with the TRIPS Agreement that allows WTO Members to authorize parallel importation, that the legislation did not address compulsory licensing, that the Minister was not granted broad powers to abrogate patent holder interests, and that, therefore, the legislation was entirely consistent with the South African Constitution. No case was brought to the WTO claiming that South Africa had breached the TRIPS Agreement.

200. In April 2001, the pharmaceutical companies in the High Court of Pretoria withdrew their suit against the government, and agreed to pay the government's legal costs in defending this case. The government reiterated its commitment to honour its obligations under the TRIPS Agreement and the companies recognized the right of South African to enact national laws or regulations, including regulations implementing the Medicines and Related Substances Control Amendment Act, in accordance with the South African Constitution and the TRIPS Agreement. The South African Government has since published for comment its proposed implementing regulations, including some that would authorize parallel importation of patented medicines.

201. Various other instances have been referred to where countries have considered that they have been under pressure from industry and/or foreign governments not to

avail themselves fully of the flexibility provided in the TRIPS Agreement. These matters have not been brought to the WTO. However, it should be noted in this connection that Article 1.1 of the TRIPS Agreement explicitly states that Members may "but shall not be obliged to" implement in their law more extensive protection than is required by the Agreement. One of the preambular provisions of the TRIPS Agreement emphasizes "the importance of reducing tensions by reaching strengthened commitments to resolve disputes on trade-related intellectual property issues through multilateral procedures". Moreover, Article 23 of the WTO Dispute Settlement Understanding commits Members who believe that other Members are not living up to their TRIPS (and other WTO) obligations to seek recourse in accordance with the Dispute Settlement Understanding and not to make determinations or take action except in accordance with it.

(viii) TRIPS and access to medicines - positions taken in some other international fora

202. At its April 2001 session, the UN Commission on Human Rights adopted a resolution (2001/33) calling upon States to refrain from taking measures which would deny or limit equal access to pharmaceuticals used to treat pandemics such as HIV/AIDS. In addition, the Commission called upon States to ensure that, as members of international organizations, they apply international agreements in support of public health policies that promote access to affordable pharmaceuticals and medical technologies.

203. The World Health Assembly's annual meeting in May 2001 devoted substantial attention to lack of access to essential drugs, which has become acute in light of the devastating human and economic impact of HIV/AIDS in many countries. WHA, as WHO's governing body, adopted a resolution (WHO Medicines Strategy, 54.11) which noted that "the impact of international trade agreements on access to, or local manufacturing of, essential drugs and on the development of new drugs needs to be further evaluated." It also requested the Director General of WHO to "enhance efforts to study and report on existing and future health implications of international trade agreements in close cooperation with relevant intergovernmental organizations." In cooperation with other intergovernmental organizations, WHO will continue to provide its Member States with information about options within TRIPS for protecting public health, pursuant to previous resolutions adopted by WHO's governing body (World Health Assembly Resolutions 52.19 and 53.14).

204. In June 2001, a special session of the UN General Assembly on HIV/AIDS also addressed the role of global trade policy in affecting the availability of low-cost generic

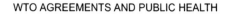

drugs and national manufacturing capacities. The special session's final declaration noted "that the impact of international trade agreements on access to or local manufacturing of, essential drugs and on the development of new drugs needs to be further evaluated."

(ix) WTO Discussions on TRIPS and access to drugs

205. At the request of the African Members of the WTO (the African Group), the TRIPS Council held a special discussion on intellectual property and access to medicines as part of its week-long regular meeting in June 2001. This was the first time that this matter had been put on the agenda of on WTO body. The work that subsequently took place in the Council for TRIPS fed into the preparatory work for the WTO Ministerial Conference held in Doha, Qatar in November 2001 and into the Declaration on the TRIPS Agreement and Public Health that was adopted by consensus by the WTO Ministers at that Conference.

206. The text of this Declaration can be found in Box 18. Its aim is to respond to the concerns expressed about the possible implications of the TRIPS Agreement for access to drugs. It does so in a number of ways. First, it emphasizes that the TRIPS Agreement does not and should not prevent Members from taking measures to protect public health and reaffirms the right of Members to use, to the full, the provisions of the TRIPS Agreement which provide flexibility for this purpose. These important declarations signal an acceptance by all WTO Members that they will not seek to prevent other Members from using these provisions.

207. Second, the Declaration makes it clear that the TRIPS Agreement should be interpreted and implemented in a manner supportive of WTO Members' right to protect public health and, in particular, to promote access to medicines for all. Further, it highlights the importance of the objectives and principles of the TRIPS Agreement for the interpretation of its provisions. Although the Declaration does not refer specifically to Articles 7 and 8 of the TRIPS Agreement, entitled, respectively, "Objectives" and "Principles", it should be noted that developing country Members attach particular importance to these provisions. These statements thus provide important guidance to both individual Members and, in the event of disputes, WTO dispute settlement bodies.

208. Third, the Declaration contains a number of important clarifications of some of the flexibilities contained in the TRIPS Agreement, while maintaining Members' commitments in the TRIPS Agreement. Details have been given in paragraphs 183 to 185 above.

209. With regard to the least-developed country Members of the WTO, the Declaration accords them an extension of their transition period until the beginning of 2016 for the protection and enforcement of patents and rights in undisclosed information with respect to pharmaceutical products. Until then, these countries are exempt from these TRIPS obligations.

210. As indicated in paragraph 184, the TRIPS Council has been mandated to find an expeditious solution to the problem of WTO Members with limited manufacturing capacities in making effective use of compulsory licencing and to report to the General Council before the end of 2002.

211. It should also be noted that, while emphasizing the scope in the TRIPS Agreement for measures to promote access to medicines, the Declaration also recognizes the importance of intellectual property protection for the development of new medicines and reaffirms the commitments of WTO Members in the TRIPS Agreement.

Box 18
Declaration on the TRIPS Agreement and public health
Adopted on 14 November 2001

1.   We recognize the gravity of the public health problems afflicting many developing and least-developed countries, especially those resulting from HIV/AIDS, tuberculosis, malaria and other epidemics.

2.   We stress the need for the WTO Agreement on Trade-Related Aspects of Intellectual Property Rights (TRIPS Agreement) to be part of the wider national and international action to address these problems.

3.   We recognize that intellectual property protection is important for the development of new medicines. We also recognize the concerns about its effects on prices.

4.   We agree that the TRIPS Agreement does not and should not prevent Members from taking measures to protect public health. Accordingly, while reiterating our commitment to the TRIPS Agreement, we affirm that the Agreement can and should be interpreted and implemented in a manner supportive of WTO Members' right to protect public health and, in particular, to promote access to medicines for all.

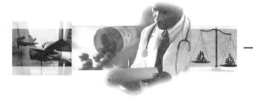

Box 18
Declaration on the TRIPS Agreement and public health
Adopted on 14 November 2001 (cont'd)

In this connection, we reaffirm the right of WTO Members to use, to the full, the provisions in the TRIPS Agreement, which provide flexibility for this purpose.

5.   Accordingly and in the light of paragraph 4 above, while maintaining our commitments in the TRIPS Agreement, we recognize that these flexibilities include:

(a) In applying the customary rules of interpretation of public international law, each provision of the TRIPS Agreement shall be read in the light of the object and purpose of the Agreement as expressed, in particular, in its objectives and principles.

(b) Each Member has the right to grant compulsory licences and the freedom to determine the grounds upon which such licences are granted.

(c) Each Member has the right to determine what constitutes a national emergency or other circumstances of extreme urgency, it being understood that public health crises, including those relating to HIV/AIDS, tuberculosis, malaria and other epidemics, can represent a national emergency or other circumstances of extreme urgency.

(d) The effect of the provisions in the TRIPS Agreement that are relevant to the exhaustion of intellectual property rights is to leave each Member free to establish its own regime for such exhaustion without challenge, subject to the MFN and national treatment provisions of Articles 3 and 4.

6.   We recognize that WTO Members with insufficient or no manufacturing capacities in the pharmaceutical sector could face difficulties in making effective use of compulsory licensing under the TRIPS Agreement. We instruct the Council for TRIPS to find an expeditious solution to this problem and to report to the General Council before the end of 2002.

7.   We reaffirm the commitment of developed-country Members to provide incentives to their enterprises and institutions to promote and encourage technology transfer to least-developed country Members pursuant to Article 66.2. We also agree that the least-developed country Members will not be obliged, with respect to pharmaceutical products, to implement or apply Sections 5 and 7 of Part II of the TRIPS Agreement or to enforce rights provided for under these Sections until 1 January 2016, without prejudice to the right of least-developed country Members to seek other extensions of the transition periods as provided for in Article 66.1 of the TRIPS Agreement. We instruct the Council for TRIPS to take the necessary action to give effect to this pursuant to Article 66.1 of the TRIPS Agreement.

212. This landmark declaration, which affirms that the TRIPS should be interpreted and implemented so as to protect public health and promote access to medicines for all, demonstrates that a rules-based trading system is compatible with public health interests. The careful and systematic attention which WTO Members afforded to fine-tuning the balance that needs to be found in the intellectual property system is indicative of the prominence accorded to public health on the international trade agenda. The declaration enshrines the principle that WHO has publicly advocated and advanced over the last four years, namely, the re-affirmation of the right of WTO Members to make full use of the safeguard provisions of the TRIPS Agreement in order to protect public health and promote access to medicines.

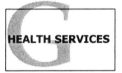

G. HEALTH SERVICES

(i) The issues

213. The equitable and efficient delivery of quality health services in response to the health needs of a population depends on many factors, including the appropriate combination of resources available on domestic as well as international markets. Ensuring that services meet the needs and expectations of the people depends on national governments setting the rules for the entire health system - what has been called responsible "stewardship" (WHO, 2000). Besides essential drugs and medical supplies as just discussed, there are several other critical resources, including qualified health personnel, well-equipped facilities, and fair financing whether through insurance coverage or affordable public sector provision.

214. International trade in health services is growing in many areas. Health professionals are moving to other countries, whether on a temporary or permanent basis, usually in search of higher wages and better working conditions. There have also been notable increases in foreign investment by hospital operators and health insurance companies in search of new markets. In addition, growing numbers of countries are seeking to attract health consumers from other countries.

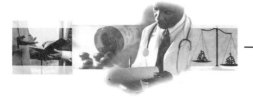

(ii) Trade in health services provides opportunities

215. Depending on appropriate regulatory conditions, trade liberalization can contribute to enhancing quality and efficiency of supplies and/or increasing foreign exchange earnings. For example, hospitals financed by foreign investors can provide certain services not previously available. New hospitals can also offer attractive employment alternatives for health professionals who might otherwise leave the country. The possible benefits resulting from health care internationalization and trade liberalization can be directed toward public health objectives in various ways. The revenue generated through the treatment of foreign patients may be used, for instance, to upgrade facilities that benefit the resident population as well. In a few developing countries, such as Thailand and Jordan, the health sector serves as a regional supply centre that attracts foreign patients who can contribute to domestic income and employment. Some developing countries, notably Cuba, India and the Philippines, "export" their doctors and nurses, producing foreign exchange remittances and filling supply gaps in host countries.

216. Health services have been listed by the WTO Secretariat among those services sectors, in which developing countries - particularly those located in the vicinity of major "markets" - may be able to benefit significantly from mode-2 trade, i.e. from attracting foreign patients (Job No. 2748/Rev.1 of 7.06.99). The 1998 UNCTAD/WHO study observed that developing countries were evolving strategies to promote such trade (p. 3). The World Bank in its 2001 publication on "Global Economic Prospects" found that health services are an area in which certain developing countries already have or could have a comparative advantage (p. 76). It is thus not surprising that in the context of the current services round, several developing countries called attention to health services liberalization under the GATS; particular reference was also made to mode-4 trade (movement of natural persons) and the possibility of creating "win-win scenarios" benefitting all countries involved (WTO documents S/CSS/M/7 of 02.03.01 and S/CSS/M/8 of 14.05.01).[62]

(iii) ... but there are risks

217. While these trends hold economic development promise, not all countries may be well-positioned to turn the potential gains into health benefits for the majority of people. Trade in health services carries risks and in some cases, has exacerbated existing problems with access and equity of health services and financing, especially for poor

---

62. The importance of services liberalization for developing countries, in particular with regard to the movement of natural persons, has recently also been stressed by the United Nations Economic Commission for Africa in its recent publication "Africa and the Multilateral Trading System and the World Trade Organization (WTO)", Addis Ababa, p. 30.

people in developing countries (UNCTAD and WHO, 1998). For example, a rise in the "brain-drain" of health professionals leaving low-income countries to work in higher-income countries, can increase health personnel shortages in developing countries, leading to problems in access to and quality of health services. It also results in losses to governments with respect to the investment made on training health professionals. The loss on investment from doctors who subsequently emigrated has been estimated at tens of millions of dollars for South Africa alone (Bundred and Levitt, 2000).[63] Developing countries that expend resources on the treatment of foreign patients may divert resources that could instead fill domestic supply needs. For-profit private, foreign-invested hospitals tend to target more lucrative markets and disregard the needs of remote regions and disadvantaged groups. In addition, by offering more attractive employment conditions, they exacerbate shortages of skilled staff in public facilities, on which the poor rely.[64] Regulatory strategies could be used to reduce such risks, but, as pointed out elsewhere, governments need to be able to enforce an effective regulatory framework for the private actors involved in health services trade (UNCTAD/WHO, 1998, p. 53).

(iv) GATS Commitments

218. The General Agreement on Trade in Services (GATS) leaves countries the flexibility to manage trade in health services in ways that are consistent with national health policy objectives (see Adlung and Carzaniga, 2001 for more details)[65]. As explained in Chapter II, countries can choose to make commitments only in some sectors and can set the limits as required to deal with various policy concerns. Although commitments are legally binding guarantees of access, governments may modify or withdraw them, subject to compensation, three years after their entry into force. Governments maintain, of course, the ability to introduce regulations in the pursuit of quality and other domestic policy objectives.

219. **Cross-border supply of health services (mode 1):** The possibility of providing certain health services across distance and, by implication, across national borders, is closely related to the advent of new communication technologies. While tele-health services were largely unknown 10 or 15 years ago, they may now be used to substitute or complement the local provision of a limited number of medical or hospital services.

63. Bundred, P.E., Levitt, C. Medical migration: who are the real losers? The Lancet, 365: 245-246. However, as explained below (para. 237), there is nothing in GATS that would prevent the "exporting" country from taking measures to stem the brain drain.

64. The existence of additional employment alternatives in new hospitals may prompt skilled staff not to move abroad.

65. Adlung, R., Carzaniga, A. Health Services under the General Agreement on Trade in Services, Bulletin of the World Health Organization, 2001, 79(4): 352-364.

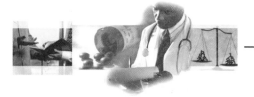

220. Nevertheless, both the novelty of the concept and concerns about appropriate regulatory enforcement may have caused many Members not to undertake commitments under this mode. In the four relevant health services sectors included in Table 1, the share of non-bindings ("unbound") is higher for mode 1 than for any other mode. For example, half of the 50-odd commitments made on medical and dental services fall within this category.

221. **Consumption of health services abroad (mode 2):** Health service exports, via the treatment of foreign patients entering their territory (mode 2), are considered and used by some countries as an instrument of economic development. A growing number of lower-income countries seek to specialize in traditional medicine and/or rely on their price competitiveness vis-à-vis higher-income countries. At the same time, many suppliers in high-income countries seek to provide more sophisticated high-tech services to patients, domestic and foreign. However, in both situations, trade opportunities are affected by trade or health-related policies in the home countries of the patients. In other words, countries that want to attract foreign patients would seek commitments under mode 2 from other countries.

222. More than half of all mode-2 commitments on medical and dental services, hospital services and other human health services are without limitations.[66] These high shares may reflect, to some extent, Members' view of consumption abroad as a possible response to a shortage in domestic health service capacity. Also, governments may have felt that their ability to prevent nationals from leaving the country and consuming services abroad is limited in any event. Without complementary domestic policies, especially portability of insurance coverage for services received abroad, consumption abroad remains an option only for well-to-do patients.

223. **Commercial Presence (mode 3):** A world-wide trend toward increased private-sector involvement in health services and health insurance has in some countries been accompanied by increasing presence of foreign investment, including in the form of joint ventures. To the extent that countries want to encourage foreign investment in the health sector, GATS commitments in mode 3 (commercial presence) are an interesting option.

224. Over 40 WTO Members have scheduled GATS commitments in mode 3 for the hospital services sub-sector, often subject to limitations which may be sector-specific

---

[66.] "Other human health services" include ambulance services, residential health facilities services other than hospital services, and services in fields such as bacteriology, virology and immunology.

(close to 30 cases) or horizontal (less than 10). It is reasonable to assume that these commitments are mostly in line with status quo conditions, rather than liberalizing market access or national treatment. Moreover, it may be worth mentioning that about 80 WTO Members have made market access commitments relating to foreign commercial presence by health insurance companies, through sectoral commitments in financial services covering the relevant subsectors. The vast majority of such commitments are partial commitments, mostly indicating limits on the number of operators or types of legal establishment that are admitted in the market. It does not appear that these commitments represent an explicit effort to encourage investment by foreign health insurers; rather, health insurance is covered as part of an overall approach to scheduling commitments on insurance.

225. **Movement of natural persons (mode 4):** Commitments on mode 4 apply to measures governing the supply of services by foreign natural persons within the relevant Members' jurisdiction. An Annex to the GATS clarifies that the Agreement does not apply to measures governments may want to use to restrict access for foreigners that seek employment, citizenship or residence on a permanent basis. If foreign health workers are seen as a desirable way to alleviate health professional shortages and/or attract new expertise and skills, countries might undertake GATS commitments under this mode.

226. To date, most GATS mode 4 commitments have remained very limited in breadth and depth. There is evidence in may cases that actual policies provide better access conditions for foreign health professionals than those bound under the GATS. So far, close to 50 Members have made partial commitments for medical and dental services and less than 30 for midwife services under mode 4. As noted before, a partial commitment means that the country concerned has reserved the right to place specified limitations on those who seek access. In turn, this increases the predictability of restrictions the country may elect to operate. In current schedules, no WTO Member has made a full commitment on health services in mode 4, probably because countries want to maintain the flexibility to decide, depending on the limitations made, on the number, type, and professional specialization of foreign personnel allowed to work in the country.

227. Overall, it appears that the commitments undertaken for hospital services carry less stringent limitations, and are thus "more liberal", than those made for the other

health services. This can be observed for developing as well as developed economies. For example, the following Members have undertaken full commitments on market access for mode 3 in this sector: Burundi, Ecuador, Kyrgyz Republic, Malawi, Swaziland, Denmark, Germany, Greece, Ireland and the United Kingdom. The commitments for the latter five countries, covered by the Schedule for the European Communities, are, however, subject to a cross-sectoral limitation indicating the non-coverage of services considered as public utilities; these may be subject to public monopolies or to exclusive rights. Other large economies with commitments in this sector include the United States and Japan. With the exception of two subsequent accessions (Ecuador and Kyrgyz Republic), the commitments have been applied since the entry into force of the GATS, i.e. January 1995 or, depending on domestic ratification procedures, some months later.

Table 1
WTO Members' commitments on medical, hospital and other health services, and on health insurance (number of Members), 3rd Quarter 2000

		Medical and Dental Services	Midwife and Nursing Services	Hospital services	Other Human Health Service	Health Insurance (in Financial Services)*	
TOTAL		52	28	42	15	78	
MARKET ACCESS							
Mode 1	Full	16 (-2)	7 (-1)	13	7	10	
	Partial	10	4	0	1	59	
	Unbound	26	17	29	7	31	
Mode 2	Full	28 (-3)	9 (-1)	36	9	22	
	Partial	22	19	4	5	52	
	Unbound	2	0	2	1	26	
Mode 3	Full	15 (-7)	5 (-2)	15 (-7)	9 (-4)	9	
	Partial	31	22	25	6	88	
	Unbound	6	1	2	0	3	
Mode 4	Full	0	0	0	0	0	
	Partial	47	27	39	15	92	
	Unbound	5	1	3	0	8	

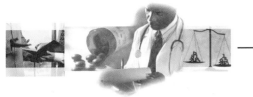

Table 1
WTO Members' commitments on medical, hospital and other health srvices, and on health insurance (number of Members), 3rd Quarter 2000 (cont'd)

		Medical and Dental Services	Midwife and Nursing Services	Hospital services	Other Human Health Service	Health Insurance (in Financial Services)*
NATIONAL TREATMENT						
Mode 1	Full	19	7	16	8	29
	Partial	8	4	0	1	32
	Unbound	25	17	26	6	39
Mode 2	Full	27 (-1)	9	36 (-1)	9 (-1)	42
	Partial	21	19	4	5	26
	Unbound	4	0	2	1	32
Mode 3	Full	17	8	29 (-23)	7 (-4)	29
	Partial	30	19	10	7	62
	Unbound	5	1	3	1	9
Mode 4	Full	1	0	2 (-1)	0	6
	Partial	47	27	37	15	82
	Unbound	4	1	3	0	12

*   *In a few cases, Members may have specifically excluded health insurance from coverage under their insurance-related commitments, but this has not yet been tabulated.*

<u>Source</u>:   WTO, 2000.

<u>Note</u>:   EC Member States are counted individually.

( ) Reduced number of full commitments if horizontal limitations are taken into account.

(v) Effects of country GATS Commitments on health services

228. What have been the effects of GATS commitments in the health service or insurance sectors? Nearly all information to date suggests that current patterns and levels of health services trade are occurring irrespective of GATS. Nor is it evident that foreign investment by health insurance companies has been influenced by GATS commitments in

the financial services sector, which often cover health insurance. There is no empirical evidence in any service sector, "to link any significant increase in FDI flows to developing countries with the conclusion of GATS" (Mashayekhi, 2000).[67] This may be due to the relatively short time that has elapsed since the conclusion of the GATS negotiations. More important, the relatively small effect so far is likely to be attributable to country commitments that bind existing levels of market access, rather than involving any substantial liberalization.

229. The overall effect of GATS on trade in health services is thus likely to have remained negligible to date. As in many other sectors, its main effect has been to make national policies more predictable in those sectors that have been subject to commitments. Measuring the effect of GATS commitments or other trade liberalization measures in individual countries is also complicated by the lack of systematic data collection over time and the difficulty of isolating the effect of trade policy on health services and systems from other changes in health care markets and in national health regulations that may occur simultaneously.

(vi) The exception for governmental services ("carve-out")

230. As already noted above, public services, that is services provided in the exercise of governmental authority, are exempt from the scope of the GATS, and thus from its rules and disciplines. This exemption applies to services that are provided neither on a commercial basis nor in competition. It is clear that in those sectors governments will be unable to undertake commitments.

231. If private and governmental services coexist in the same jurisdiction, governments can still consider commitments on the former. This is reflected, for example, in the European Communities' Schedule which explicitly excludes from coverage all services provided by public utilities. If these utilities provide governmental services within the meaning of Article I:3, this limitation may not even be necessary as the Article would apply in any event. Concern has been expressed that the co-existence of private and governmental services, regardless of the existence of commitments, affects the application of the governmental-service carve-out. In nearly all countries, public sector health providers co-exist with private health providers and the two commonly provide similar services, and patients move abroad for treatment in foreign hospitals. Does this entail "competition"? In most countries, public-sector health providers charge user fees

[67]. Mashayekhi, M. GATS 2000 Negotiations: Options for Developing Countries: A Positive Agenda for Developing Countries: Issues for Future Trade Negotiations, UNCTAD (Document No.UNCTAD/ITCD/TSB/10), 2000.

to patients. Does this make the provision of the services "commercial"? Because none of these issues has yet resulted in a dispute between WTO Members, there is no definitive interpretation and, as noted above, while WTO Member governments could seek clarification within the current GATS negotiations, they have not yet expressed the need to do so. This may have something to do with the fact that, for a country that has not committed on health services, the application, or not, of the governmental services carve-out would not have market access or national treatment implications, but merely determine the applicability of the MFN principle and some procedural obligations (related to transparency for example). Non-application of the carve-out would imply that the MFN requirement comes into play, meaning that all existing and any new trade restrictions would have to be applied vis-à-vis all WTO Members.

(vii) Trade liberalization as a risk to quality, equity and other public policy objectives?

232. There is a concern that opening health markets to foreign competition poses risks to equity, access and quality of services available to the poor. Some evidence indicates that benefits of opening markets are concentrated among the wealthy. For example, a multinational investment fund that has invested in several Latin American managed care companies and acquired public hospital management contracts, has sought to reduce the proportion of uninsured patients in its hospitals (Stocker, et.al, 1999)[68]. A potential benefit of foreign direct investment is that it may provide high-quality services that are not currently available domestically. In the absence of government regulation, these services are, however, likely to be only available to those who can afford it.

233. Governments which make commitments to allow foreign suppliers to provide health services can enforce the same standards for the protection of the public on foreign suppliers as on nationals, and can, indeed, impose additional requirements on foreigners if they so choose. In the latter case, a national treatment limitation would need to be scheduled. To increase potential benefits of foreign direct investments for the population at large, governments can, for instance, with regard to private health insurance, require all private insurance plans - foreign and domestically-owned - to offer a basic package of benefits, prohibit "dumping" of high-cost patients onto the public system, and prohibit the exclusion of people with pre-existing conditions and diseases. In addition, governments can require private health providers to provide a certain amount of free care to the poor, or tax the facilities and dedicate the revenue to support public health services. To limit any reduction in health service capacity for dis-

68. Stocker, K., Waitzkin, H., Iriart, C. Health Policy Report: The Exportation of Managed Care to Latin America, The New England Journal of Medicine, April 8, 1999, Vol. 340, No. 14: 1131-1136.

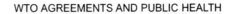

advantaged groups, a government may require private hospitals, for example, to:
(a) reserve a minimum percentage of beds for free treatment to the needy; (b) offer some basic medical services in remote rural areas; or (c) train a higher number of staff than required for their own purposes.

234. Turning to exports of health services (those provided to foreigners), the GATS does not impose constraints on the terms and conditions on which a host country treats foreigners consuming services within its territory: any restrictions on the services provided to tourists or foreign patients are beyond the Agreement's scope. WTO Members thus remain free to subject such services to quotas, taxes or charges, and to use any proceeds to enhance the quantity and/or quality of basic health services.

235. While liberalization (at home or abroad) might increase the outflow of qualified staff from the public sector to the private sector (at home or abroad), there are no legal impediments in the GATS on governments' rights to discourage such movements of personnel. To lessen the costs of the brain drain, countries might consider a variety of measures that would help to compensate for the loss of trained health professionals. Countries could levy taxes on those who leave the country, or require deposits or financial guarantees, with the costs borne by the countries or private organizations that do the recruiting. In addition, there are "positive" measures that might limit the risk of a "brain drain", for example enhanced career development opportunities and conditions of employment; foreign investment in a country's hospital sector, possibly combined with inflows of foreign patients, might also enhance domestic employment opportunities and, in turn, dissuade staff from leaving.

(viii) GATS recognizes the right to regulate

236. The preamble of the GATS Agreement expressly "recognizes the rights of Members to regulate, and to introduce new regulations, on the supply of services within their territories in order to meet national policy objectives ... ". Countries without commitments in the health sector or the health insurance sub-sectors are free to adopt any policies, regardless of their effects on trade, with the main binding constraint being the MFN principle. It requires that regulations must not discriminate between like **foreign** services or service suppliers of different origin or nationality. In sectors where Members have scheduled full commitments on national treatment, they are obliged not to discriminate against foreign services or service suppliers in their regulations, but are, of

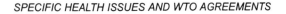

course, still free to regulate the sector to meet public policy objectives. If a country wishes to reserve the right to apply more stringent rules to foreign services or suppliers than to national ones, these rules would need to be covered by limitations on national treatment in its schedule.

(ix) . . . but regulatory capacity may be weak or non-existent in some developing countries

237. While GATS gives governments a wide scope to regulate private health providers and insurers to protect equity, such regulations may be weak or non-existent in a number of developing countries. According to the WHO, as of the mid-1990s, "with a few notable exceptions (Hungary, Colombia), there are, for instance, virtually no comprehensive regulations for health insurance. Moreover, where there are regulations on the books, enforcement is often limited or ineffective "(Chollet and Lewis, 1997).[69] This may equally be true in certain cases of the regulation of health facilities, professionals and services. Until regulatory systems are in place and the capacity to implement them is strengthened, there is a risk that suppliers will compromise efforts to achieve equity in access or financing, or engage in consumer fraud, although publicly owned and operated facilities are not immune from regulatory failure or negligence either. Strengthened regulation may be a precondition in a number of countries for liberalization to be consistent with health sector objectives. This is a challenging task, especially for those developing countries whose regulatory systems have limited human and financial resources. The possibility of undertaking pre-commitments, i.e. commitments that apply only years after the conclusion of the new round (see paragraph 81 above), may help to provide the time needed for careful regulatory reform. The countries concerned may also benefit from joining forces, seeking synergies or working with relevant international organisations to strengthen capacity in this area.

(x) Liberalization calls for greater regulation

238. The need to regulate the private sector typically increases as competing suppliers enter the market. Governments need to act to prevent any adverse effects and channel any gains to benefit health. Greater, not less, regulation has accompanied more open markets in financial services and telecommunications, and this will be essential for health services as well. Thus, the tasks of Ministries of Health will likely increase if health services trade is liberalized, making it critical for them to advise Ministries of Trade on the effects of opening up their health systems to competition.

---

69. Chollet, D., Lewis, M. Private Insurance: Principles and Practice, Paper presented at the Conference on Innovations in Health Care Financing, sponsored by the World Bank, 10-11 March 1997, Washington DC.

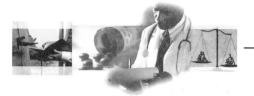

(xi) The on-going GATS negotiations provide an opportunity for input

239. Ministries of Trade and Health in all countries have an interest in closely following current GATS negotiations. The negotiations, which began in 2000, are expected to widen the sector coverage of current schedules and deepen the level of existing commitments. At the time of writing, health was the only large service sector that has eluded specific proposals for liberalization. Nevertheless, the negotiations are a source of concern to some public health advocates, who fear that they will prompt governments to open up their publicly funded health services to private, for-profit foreign investors.

240. The Guidelines and Procedures for the Negotiations on Trade in Services, agreed by Members in March 2001, state that "the process of liberalization shall take place with due respect for national policy objectives, the level of development and the size of economies of individual Members, both overall and in individual sectors". There is no obligation on any WTO Member to allow foreign supply of any particular service, nor even to guarantee domestic competition. Nor has the GATS any implications for the funding of services provided in the exercise of governmental authority. Also, the structure and content of the GATS Article XIX guarantees developing countries "appropriate flexibility ... for opening fewer sectors, liberalizing fewer types of transactions, and progressively extending market access in line with their development situation".

241. Even if countries choose not to liberalize trade in the health sector in the current round of negotiations, measures in other sectors can be relevant to health: For example, education commitments that affect the training of, and thus the scope of employment possibilities for, medical and health professionals; or commitments leading to improved transport and communication systems; or commitments in environmental or financial services. On a more general level, income effects generated by a more liberal trading environment can have positive effects on health through a variety of channels, such as increased government resources available for public health measures or increased household incomes spent on personal health care.

242. Some WTO Members have submitted proposals that would facilitate the application of existing commitments on movements of natural persons (e.g. through clarification of the terms and definitions used in schedules) and foresee the negotiation of new commitments. It may need to be reiterated that such commitments apply only to the access conditions offered by the (potential) host countries and do not affect in any way

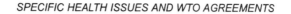

the possibility of the originating countries to regulate (temporary) outflows of their residents. For example, a requirement on newly trained staff to work first for some time in domestic facilities, rather than capitalizing abroad on taxpayers' investment in their education, would be perfectly compatible with the GATS and any commitments undertaken in schedules.

243. WHO is undertaking to monitor GATS Council debates and proposals, assess their health implications, and disseminate information to the public. Upon request of Member States, WHO will also help country health officials evaluate GATS commitments, assess which limitations are important to ensure they are consistent with health policies and public health objectives, and analyze the impact of existing or potential trade liberalization policies on the health sector. The WTO Secretariat also responds to any questions concerning the interpretation of GATS provisions and their relevance for individual services sectors. The Trade in Services Division frequently conducts country missions to inform officials from interested ministries and agencies of the structure of the Agreement and its relevance to individual sectors; ways and means of pursuing sector-specific objectives in a GATS-consistent way; interpreting the commitments scheduled by other Members; and the state of play in the ongoing services negotiations. Relevant information, including on all negotiating proposals obtained to date, is available on the WTO website.

244. In sum, the commitment to progressive liberalization presents a potential for negotiating expanded commitments on trade in health services and, by the same token, an opportunity to attract foreign direct investment and make it responsive to national health priorities. In many developing countries, this offers opportunities to acquire health services unavailable domestically or export health services and human resources to a larger world market. At the same time, there are risks of exacerbating existing problems of access and equity of health services and financing. The challenge is to maximize the opportunities and minimize the risks. Trade liberalization heightens the need for effective regulatory frameworks to ensure that private sector activity in the health system generates the expected benefits. Each country will assess the relevant implications in developing its negotiating stance in GATS negotiations and is free to decide whether to liberalize any given service, and if so, in what way and at what pace.

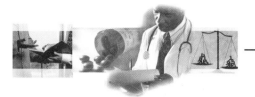

FOOD SECURITY AND NUTRITION

H. FOOD SECURITY AND NUTRITION

(i) Nutrition and health

245. Malnutrition or under-nutrition (inadequate calorie intake relative to needs) is responsible for an estimated 16 per cent of the global burden of disease, and about a third of the burden of disease in Sub-Saharan Africa (Murray and Lopez, 1996)[70]. It increases the risk of communicable and non-communicable diseases, and worsens the prognosis when such diseases are contracted. In pregnant women, it increases the risk of obstetric complications, maternal mortality, low-birth weight babies and infant morbidity and mortality. Childhood under-nutrition, leading to stunting, increases health risks later in life. Access to relatively high energy-density foods (e.g. dairy products, oils and fats) is particularly important to childhood nutrition during weaning. Further health problems arise from inadequate intakes of protein, vitamins and minerals, especially in children, e.g. anaemia (iron), adverse outcomes from measles (vitamin A), and bone weakness (calcium and vitamin D).

(ii) Food security and nutrition

246. The Rome Declaration on World Food Security states that:

"Food security exists when all people, at all times, have physical and economic access to sufficient, safe and nutritious food to meet their dietary needs and food preferences for an active and healthy life."

247. Food security[71] is generally considered at two levels:

(a) **National food security** is the ability of a country to secure an adequate *total supply* of food to meet the nutritional needs of its population at all times, through domestic production, food imports and/or the temporary use of national food stocks.

(b) **Household food security** is the ability of a household to secure reliable *access* to enough food for its members at all times, through its own production (subsistence), market purchases, use of its own stocks and/or public provision.

[70]. Murray, J.L., Lopez, A.D. (eds.). The Global Burden of Disease. World Health Organization/Harvard School of Public Health/World Bank, 1996.

[71]. Food security should not be confused with food safety, which is discussed earlier in this report (page 58).

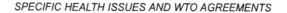
248. The issue of food security is complex and has many components. At the national level, economic access to food is critically dependent on national production and distribution, access to international markets and the availability of foreign exchange to buy imports. At the household level, it is dependent on the level and stability of household incomes and food production for own consumption, savings, access to credit, and the prices of food and other essential goods. At both levels, physical access is critically dependent on peace, security and reliable transportation. Taken together, these challenges are formidable by any standard, and addressing them effectively requires action at both the national and the international level. Trade policies are only one factor in the equation.

249. While the health effects of food insecurity are most apparent in the context of famines - that is, of an acute failure of national food security - the great majority of the burden of disease associated with undernutrition arises from chronic malnutrition as a result of *household* food insecurity. This is affected by economic and social policies at home. It is also affected by trade liberalization through a number of different impacts on household incomes and employment opportunities and on prices of foods and other essentials. These impacts are both direct and indirect (e.g. operating through national economic performance and international markets). Because of its complexity, household food security is not discussed in this report, despite its central importance to the burden of disease. The following discussion therefore focuses only on national food security.

(iii) Trade liberalization and national food security ...

250. National food security is a concern primarily in countries which rely on imports of basic foods. In such countries, trade liberalization may reduce self-sufficiency in basic food production and increase reliance on imports. However, this is not the same as worsening national food security, which is affected primarily by a country's ability to earn enough foreign exchange to import the food it needs.

251. Export agriculture remains a cornerstone of the economies of many developing countries and is the main source of foreign exchange for many low-income countries. Agricultural trade liberalization helps to improve their export growth, including by creating opportunities for developing non-traditional exports, e.g. fruit, vegetables or cut flowers, thus providing more foreign exchange with which to import essential imports

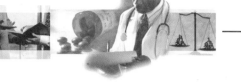

into agricultural production as well as food. If trade barriers are lowered more for processed than for unprocessed products, this might also encourage the development of processing industries and increase the value-added of exports. Likewise, lower trade barriers for labour-intensive manufactures could generate new export opportunities, e.g. for textiles, leather goods and wood products. It is therefore no surprise that developing countries have been very active, for instance, in the on-going WTO negotiations on agriculture.

252. By reducing export subsidies as well as subsidies linked to production and by lowering trade barriers, trade liberalization may, at least in the short term, reduce supply and increase demand, thus raising world food prices, particularly for cereals and temperate crops. Least-developed and net food-importing developing countries have therefore been concerned about the impact on their food import bills. On average, food imports represent about 16 per cent of total imports of least-developed countries, and 11 per cent for net food-importing developing countries, although this varies enormously from one country to another, with figures up to 30-40 per cent in some of the latter group (FAO, Agricultural Trade Database). Cereals account for some 40 per cent of food imports in these countries as a whole, and oils and fats for a further 20 per cent.

253. In principle, the benefits of trade liberalization in terms of improved market access have the potential to offset the costs of higher world food prices. Moreover, to the extent that the price distortions on the world market are eliminated, this would provide an additional benefit for developing country exporters of the products concerned and also stimulate agricultural development in those net food-importing developing countries where depressed world food prices and subsidized import competition have adversely affected domestic production. These effects may not come about everywhere and not necessarily in the short-term, due in part to supply side constraints, limited opening of developed country markets, or difficulties in meeting the sanitary and phytosanitary standards applied by developed countries. There are also concerns that further trade liberalization will erode existing trade preferences. At the same time, however, it opens up new access opportunities in non-preferential markets, an important point not least because south-south trade in agricultural products has been growing and today already accounts for around 40 per cent of developing country agricultural exports.

254. Increased reliance on imports of basic foods increases vulnerability to international market conditions, especially commodity price fluctuations, as well as threats to

physical access to food (e.g. conflict or other adverse conditions in neighbouring countries for land-locked countries). However, that risk has to be compared with the risks of a closed economy where domestic supply of food is, amongst other things, at the mercy of the weather. In any event, if trade liberalization of countries facing food insecurity is not mirrored by liberalization in their export markets, they will need to sell more of their existing exports - notably tropical agricultural products - to pay for additional food imports without a corresponding increase in world demand, and the resulting increase in supply could exacerbate the long-term decline in export prices.

255. A major concern for developing countries is thus the level of agricultural support and protection that remains in the developed world and which has not, in their eyes, resulted in anything close to a "level playing field". The need for improved market access is a major issue. Tariff peaks and tariff escalation (higher tariff rates on processed than unprocessed products) in developed countries are important obstacles to adding value to agricultural products and diversifying production. At the same time, trade-distorting subsidies provided by trading partners further undermine domestic food production, and, since developing countries cannot compete with the scale of subsidies in the developed world, some which have the potential to be food exporters are instead net importers.

(iv) Food aid

256. Food aid is important in limiting the effects of national food insecurity, especially in emergency situations. However, it is essential to minimize any adverse impacts of food aid on agricultural development in recipient countries. Under WTO rules, food aid is exempted from export subsidy reduction commitments, but only subject to certain conditions, including the requirement for food-aid transactions to be in accordance with the FAO Principles of Surplus Disposal and Consultative Obligations.[72] Furthermore, public holding of food stocks for food security purposes is excluded from the WTO Agreement on Agriculture restrictions on production subsidies, provided that they are conducted through a publicly funded government programme, that they do not have the effect of providing price support to producers, and that all purchases are at market prices. This leaves governments free to pursue such policies, subject only to their own resource constraints, and the policy conditions of the international financial institutions and donors.

---

[72] The other conditions are (i) that the provision of the food aid is not tied directly or indirectly to commercial exports of agricultural products to recipient countries, and (ii) that such aid be provided to the extent possible on grant terms and at least on terms no less concessional than those provided for in Article IV of the Food Aid Convention 1986.

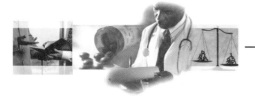

257. Food aid is also addressed in the Ministerial Decision on Measures Concerning the Possible Negative Effects of the Reform Programme on Least-Developed and Net Food-Importing Developing Countries (NFIDC Decision).[73] In accordance with this Decision, the Food Aid Convention was re-negotiated, and the new Convention came into effect on 1 July 1999.[74] This Decision also has other provisions, including a commitment by donors to give full consideration in the context of their aid programmes to requests for the provision of technical and financial assistance to least-developed and net-food importing developing countries to improve their agricultural productivity and infrastructure. On the initiative of net food-importing developing countries, which consider that it has not been adequately implemented, the Decision is one of the implementation issues currently being addressed by the General Council in the framework of the Implementation Review Mechanism.[75]

(v) The ongoing negotiations represent an opportunity

258. The ongoing WTO negotiations on agriculture represent an opportunity to advance the agricultural trade and food security agenda, and developing countries have participated actively in them. In the first phase of the negotiations, from March 2000 to March 2001, a total of 121 WTO Members tabled 45 negotiating proposals, compared with 5 proposals from 35 countries during the first year of the Uruguay Round; in the second phase, another 105 elaborated proposals, and other non-papers have been submitted by Members. These negotiations have received further direction through the mandate and the time-frames set out in the Doha Ministerial Declaration. With the adoption, in March 2002, of a detailed programme to establish modalities for the further commitments in the areas of export subsidization, market access and domestic support by March 2003, the negotiations have entered a crucial stage.

259. Food security and related issues are being addressed in several ways in these negotiations. For example, a wide range of countries have called for the elimination of export subsidies and other forms of export subsidization so as to put an end to their adverse impact on the production systems of developing countries. In addition, a group of developing countries has emphasized the need to give developing countries additional

---

[73.] In addition to all least-developed countries, the following net food-importing developing countries are currently on the WTO list related to this Decision. Barbados, Botswana, Côte d'Ivoire, Cuba, Dominica, Dominican Republic, Egypt, Honduras, Jamaica, Jordan, Kenya, Mauritius, Morocco, Pakistan, Peru, Saint Kitts and Nevis, Saint Lucia, Saint Vincent and the Grenadines, Senegal, Sri Lanka, Trinidad and Tobago, Tunisia and Venezuela (see G/AG/5/Rev.4).

[74.] For more detail, see: www.igc.org.uk

[75.] For information on the state of play in the negotiations on agriculture, including information on food-security-related negotiating proposals, see the WTO website (WTO trade topics, agriculture negotiations (www.wto.org)).

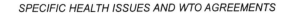

flexibilities to address their food security concerns, including flexibility to support their own production of essential food crops and for such assistance to be exempt from any reduction commitment as part of a proposed Development/Food Security Box. There have also been calls for the strengthening of the current disciplines on export restrictions to increase the reliability of global food supply, for example by preventing developed countries from taxing their food exports and thereby reducing supply on the world market when prices are high. Furthermore, proposals have been made for developed countries to make more specific commitments in respect of food aid, and a number of other concrete proposals are on the table designed to address the concerns of net food-importing developing countries.

I. EMERGING ISSUES

260. Advances in technology constitute one of the major driving forces behind globalization and international trade, as well as health improvements. But technological advances sometimes occur faster than the pace at which societies can understand or respond to their implications for public policy. Within the health arena, there are two important technological advances that have the potential to revolutionize health care - biotechnology and information technology. A third emerging health issue is related, paradoxically, to the centuries-old use of herbal medicines and traditional knowledge for treating illnesses. All three issues represent the next wave of policy issues involving health and trade.

1. Biotechnology

261. Though the range of activities that come under the term are diverse, biotechnology can be generally defined as "the application of scientific and engineering principles to the processing of materials by biological agents to provide goods and services" (OECD, 1982).[76] Biotechnology has already made enormous contributions to biomedical research and is beginning to translate into real-world applications in disease prevention and treatment. But as the scope of its application grows wider, from humans and animals to genes and viruses to plants and trees, its impact on society and on economies is also widening.

[76.] Bull, A.T., Holt, G., Lilly, M.D. International Trends and Perspectives, OECD, 1982.

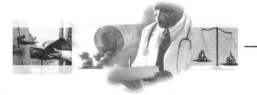
262. The fruits of biotechnological discoveries of the last 20 or so years have already led to new diagnostic tests, pharmaceuticals, and medical treatments for a long list of diseases, from diabetes (production of human insulin proteins) to molecular-based detection of tuberculosis. The recent decoding of the human genome represented the culmination of years of scientific inquiry and ushers in a new age of potential medical advances. Data on human chromosomes are already being used to investigate the genetic underpinnings of health and disease.

(i) Concern about patents

263. Like the controversy over patents on drugs or vaccines of vital public health importance, the patenting of biotechnology products raises several concerns. One set of concerns relates to the patentability of biotechnological innovations, i.e. whether they meet the basic criteria of novelty, inventiveness and usefulness. There are differences of opinion about whether data on human gene sequences should qualify for patents, even though private companies have already applied for and received patents for them. At issue here is the interpretation of the basic criteria for patentability - novelty, inventive step and industrial applicability - which have for long been found in all patent laws in both developed and developing countries (the WTO TRIPS Agreement refers to these basic criteria without further interpreting them). Some of the data on human gene sequences is already owned by private companies, which are filing patent applications despite arguments about whether the sequences should qualify for patenting. Another concern is that if patents are given to genetically modified proteins or DNA that are key active ingredients in new vaccines, it could lead to significant price increases by limiting competition to a narrow field of vaccine producers, who now usually obtain patents for the production process rather than the chemical products contained in vaccines.

264. Intellectual property issues in relation to biotechnology have been discussed within the WTO, both in the Committee on Trade and Environment and in the TRIPS Council's review of Article 27.3(b), relating to patentability of biotechnological inventions. In the TRIPS Council, the issues raised include ethical and moral questions relating to the patentability of life-forms; what qualifies as inventive; and how concrete the potential use needs to be - e.g. with respect to DNA and the genome, whether this requires that the gene's function be specified, or a commercial application related to it. In addition, there is debate surrounding the definition of certain terms in the TRIPS Agreement such as "microorganisms"; the meaning of effective sui generis protection of

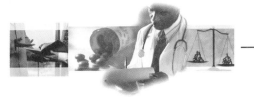

new plant varieties, including its relationship to the International Convention for the Protection of New Varieties of Plants (UPOV); the relationship between the TRIPS Agreement and the Convention on Biological Diversity; and the protection of traditional knowledge.

(ii) Food security and safety

265. Biotechnology also holds potential to make food production more efficient, contribute to increased harvests, and improve public health. For example, "Golden Rice", a genetically modified rice that produces beta-carotene which the body converts into vitamin A, may help to alleviate vitamin A deficiency, a major cause of blindness in developing countries of Africa and Asia. But there is not yet complete information on the costs and health effects of this new product compared to alternative methods to reduce blindness. This issue reflects broader safety concerns about genetically-modified foods, such as: the potential for gene transfer from genetically modified plants to microbial or mammalian cells; the transfer and expression of a functional antibiotic resistance gene to recipient cells in people or animals; and, allergenic effects.

266. National and regional regulatory systems exist to examine the safety of genetically modified foods, but there are significant differences in testing methods that produce inconsistent outcomes of safety evaluations. Efforts are under way by WHO and FAO, and the Codex Alimentarius Commission, to determine needed changes in safety assessments of genetically modified foods, and in international rules on the handling of genetically modified foods. An Inter-Agency Network for Safety in Biotechnology (IANB) was formed in 1999, in Paris at the OECD. Its objectives are to share information and to promote co-operation amongst inter-governmental agencies with activities related to safety in biotechnology.[77]

267. Despite the heated public debate in Europe and elsewhere, there has been little formal consideration of the health and safety aspects of biotechnology and GMOs in WTO fora. The most detailed discussions to date have occurred in the TBT Committee, where the GMO labelling requirements of various Members have been under scrutiny. Issues relating to food safety and to the potential spread of genetically modified seeds into the environment may fall under the SPS Agreement. The SPS Committee had discussions with respect to the negotiations of the Biosafety Protocol. The need for transparency and the development of international standards was also discussed in relation to concerns about GMO-related notifications and, in other cases, with regard to the

---

77. Participants: CGIAR, CBD, ICGEB, FAO, OIE, OECD, UNCTAD, UNDP, UNIDO, WHO and WTO (for more detail see www.oecd.org/subject/biotech).

absence of notification of measures to the WTO. Also, in the context of the ongoing agriculture negotiations, there has been a proposal to focus disciplines to ensure that processes covering trade in products developed through "new technologies" are transparent, predictable and timely. Nevertheless, there has not yet been substantive discussion of either of these proposals.

(iii) The Cartagena Biosafety Protocol

268. The Cartagena Biosafety Protocol[78] gives governments the right to prohibit imports of living modified organisms (LMOs) intended for planting or other direct release into the environment for health and environmental reasons. LMOs are basically GMOs such as seeds that have not been processed, and that could live if introduced into the environment.[79] Prior informed consent must be given before trade can take place, and precautionary prohibitions may be maintained. For products which contain living modified organisms but which are intended for direct consumption or further processing, the requirements are less onerous, but require information on GMO products to be submitted through a clearinghouse mechanism prior to trade, and again precautionary prohibitions are possible. The objective of the Protocol is to ensure an adequate level of protection in the field of safe transfer, handling and use of LMOs that may have adverse effects on the conservation and sustainable use of biological diversity, taking into account risks to human health.

269. While there is scope for complementarity between the Protocol and WTO agreements, there is also scope for inconsistencies. For example, under the Cartagena Protocol, a country which wants to export LMOs - such as seeds for planting - must seek advance informed agreement from the importing country before the first shipment takes place, and, under certain circumstances, the importer can ask the exporter to carry out the risk assessment. Under the SPS Agreement, it is up to the importer to justify its import measure on the basis of a risk assessment. Here the obligations are different. It is unclear which international agreement would rule in the event of a conflict and to what extent these apparently conflicting obligations would, in practice, be a problem. In any case, if a dispute were brought to the WTO, a panel or the Appellate Body could

78. This is a Protocol to the Convention on Biological Diversity. It was adopted in January 2000 and in June 2001 had 100 signatories. The Protocol will enter into force after 50 countries have ratified it (three countries had ratified it by June 2001).
79. The Protocol defines a "living modified organism" as "any living organism that possesses a novel combination of genetic material obtained through the use of modern biotechnology". A "living organism" is "any biological entity capable of transferring or replicating genetic material, including sterile organisms, viruses and viroids".

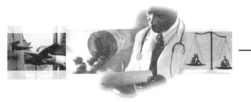

only judge compliance with WTO Agreements. Nevertheless, in doing so the Cartagena Protocol would presumably be taken into account, when the two disputing parties are also signatories of the Protocol.

2. Information technology

270. Informatics and telecommunications are transforming societies and many economies, raising job productivity, creating new jobs, and speeding up communication and information flows. This trend has already stimulated changes in health care delivery, and has the potential to foster greater cross-border supply of health services. Diagnostic and treatment services can currently be supplied across borders using telecommunications technology. For example, a patient may be seen at a video-equipped facility by a medical consultant in another country. Interpretative services, such as those related to pathology specimens and diagnostic imaging are the most immediate growth opportunity given that the transmission of static images requires far less bandwidth than video for diagnosis. In the longer term, information technology allowing real-time three-dimensional control of precision instruments with operator feedback may even support the remote performance of surgical procedures. Its use in cross-border trade to serve the poor, however, could be constrained by high cost and lack of infrastructure and trained personnel.

271. Since 1998, WTO Members have been engaged in a comprehensive work programme aimed at examining trade-related issues relative to electronic commerce. At the time the work programme was initiated, Members undertook to continue the practice of not imposing customs duties on electronic transmissions. In addition, pharmaceuticals ordered electronically, for instance, should be subject to the same border treatment, e.g. tariffs and product verification, as those ordered by regular mail. Except for protection of life or health, medical advice provided electronically from another country should be subject to the same rules as that provided by mail (Adlung and Carzaniga, 2000). Electronic commerce in health services may also have some unique problems; foreign providers' quality of care cannot be examined as easily as the quality and safety of health goods. Countries allowing such commerce might need to certify foreign telemedicine providers, which may be a burdensome task. In any event, concerns about the security and privacy of health transactions, as well as questions about legal liability and licensing requirements, are likely to play a much greater role than concerns about quality in determining the use and growth of electronic commerce in health care.

272. Taking a broader perspective, there may be opportunities for information technology to involve civil society in public policy debates on health-and-trade issues at the national level. Recent discussions of the public policy implications of information technology and the Internet promote the notion of "e-governance", which goes beyond government's role in promoting information technology for e-commerce. Governments could use information technology to create more open and transparent government processes, empower citizens to participate in policy debates, and promote development and democracy more broadly. Seen from this angle, information technology could become a powerful tool for involving civil society in deciding issues relating to national health or health-and-trade policies.

3. Protection of traditional medicine knowledge

273. The knowledge of medicinal plants and their healing properties has been built up over centuries, perhaps even millennia, and passed on between generations. Large segments of the population in the developing world continue to rely on medicinal plants while demand is growing among people in industrialized nations, contributing to growing international trade in herbal medicines. World trade in plants with medicinal value was estimated at $1.3 billion annually in 1996, growing at 10 to 20 per cent per year (Financial Times, 5 February 2000). For China, it now represents a significant source of export earnings, and for Bhutan which has the world's highest concentration of medicinal plants, it has significant potential. Countries vary in their regulatory approach to production and use of medicinal plants for health purposes (WHO, 1998).

274. As the knowledge of traditional medicine and medicinal plants grows in economic and trade value, the need to protect it and secure fair and equitable sharing of any benefits derived from it is of increasing concern. Traditional knowledge has been intensively discussed in the WTO TRIPS Council in the context of the review of Article 27.3(b) of the TRIPS Agreement, which started in 1999. Among the issues under discussion in the TRIPS Council relevant to the subject of traditional medicinal knowledge are the following:

(a) Protection of traditional knowledge either through existing forms of intellectual property rights or other laws or through a sui generis form of protection.
(b) Prevention of the improper patenting of traditional knowledge and plant genetic resources, including how to improve the databases of such knowledge for this purpose.

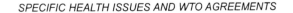

(c) The relationship between the TRIPS Agreement and the Convention on Biological Diversity in general and the operational implementation of the provisions of prior informed consent and fair and equitable benefit sharing as set out in Article 8(j) of the Convention on Biological Diversity in particular.

(d) The relation of work in the TRIPS Council with intergovernmental discussions on this issue such as in the CBD, WIPO, FAO and UNCTAD.

275. Many of these issues were discussed in a WHO workshop on intellectual property rights in the context of traditional medicine, in December 2000.[80] Other work in this area is being pursued by WIPO to explore how existing intellectual property rights can be used to provide protection to traditional medicine practitioners. Others stress the difficulties that herbal medicines and traditional medicinal practitioners will face if they rely only on Western models of intellectual property rights protection. Thus, there is a need to develop alternative approaches to promote and protect traditional medicine and assure an equitable sharing of its benefits. In addition, it will be important to explore how countries can utilize the flexibility provided under the TRIPS Agreement to promote easy access to traditional medicines for health care needs of developing countries.

276. These three issues - biotechnology, information technology, and protection of indigenous medicines and knowledge - are among several emerging health-and-trade issues. As the world becomes more integrated and inter-connected, the health issues of today can quickly become the trade issues of tomorrow and vice versa. Traditional divisions within governments between health and trade ministries no longer serve national interests, when health and trade issues converge. The usual boundaries between "health people" and "trade people" - both in national governments and in international organizations involved in health and trade - hamper better understanding of how trade and health issues affect each other. Breaking down the walls that divide the two camps thus represents one of the most important ways to solve and prevent health problems of the future, and to make faster progress towards common health and economic development goals.

---

80. Report available at: http://www.who.int/medicines/library/trm/who-edm-trm-2001-1/who-edm-trm-2001-1en.htm.

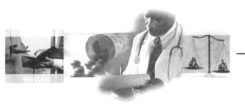

IV. TOWARDS HEALTH AND TRADE POLICY COHERENCE

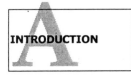

A. INTRODUCTION

277. There is common ground between health and trade, and between the objectives of the WHO and the WTO. The WHO's objective is "the attainment of all peoples of the highest possible level of health", and WHO defines health as "a state of complete physical, mental and social well-being and not merely the absence of disease or infirmity". Good health is one important building block for sustainable economic development. With regard to trade, an underlying assumption is that a liberal international trade regime, subject to reasonably stable and predictable conditions, improves the climate for investment, production and employment creation, and therefore contributes to economic growth and development. Generally, the health status of a country is affected positively by such growth. This expectation is reflected in the opening words of the agreement establishing the World Trade Organization:

"The Parties to this Agreement,
Recognizing that their relations in the field of trade and economic endeavour
should be conducted with a view to raising standards of living...."

278. As this report has shown, the rules and provisions of the WTO agreements most relevant to health generally permit countries to manage trade in goods and services in order to achieve their national health objectives, as long as health measures respect basic trade principles such as non-discrimination. Even these provisions may be waived under exceptions for public health reasons as provided in many WTO Agreements.

279. Yet concerns have been expressed by some observers that WTO rules could constitute a threat to sound public health policies. The disagreements over hormone-treated beef or, potentially, trade in genetically modified foods and recent discussions on TRIPS and access to medicines, illustrate possible tensions between national health and trade policies.

280. A constructive way to address such concerns is to view them as opportunities for finding common ground. Minimizing possible conflicts between trade and health, and

maximizing their mutual benefits, is an example of policy coherence. The term refers to efforts to seek synergies between policies in different areas in support of their common goals - in this case, poverty reduction, human development and economic growth. The need for greater policy coherence at the international level has been highlighted at several recent UN conferences, while many national governments are striving to bring foreign trade and development policies into closer alignment.

281. The final section of this report stresses the importance of the goal of coherence between health and trade policies at the national and international level. It describes efforts in two countries - Canada and Thailand - directed towards health-and-trade policy coherence at the national level. Second, it examines efforts to coordinate activities at the international level between WHO and WTO and reviews opportunities to enhance policy coherence. It concludes with suggestions for new avenues through which health, trade and development officials can pursue greater policy coherence and thus make a stronger contribution to the goal of more sustainable human and economic development.

TOWARDS POLICY
COHERENCE AT
NATIONAL AND
INTERNATIONAL
LEVELS

B. TOWARDS POLICY COHERENCE AT NATIONAL AND INTERNATIONAL LEVELS

282. Policy coherence is easy to support in principle but hard to achieve in practice. It requires regular dialogue, consultation, and coordinated action between policy-makers and advisors on all sides. Similar challenges exist, and are being addressed in other policy areas as well (trade and finance, trade and environment, for example). Two divergent perspectives underlie the interface between trade considerations and health interests. From a Trade Ministry perspective, health may be looked at in the context of trade agreements that are essentially about liberalizing trade. By contrast, health professionals may perceive that the need to submit health measures to trade scrutiny will subordinate health to trade interests. These perspectives may cause tension between "trade people" and "health people", and render coherence difficult.

283. Safeguarding health is an objective that nobody would question. In the context of the WTO, government officials involved are likely to examine carefully how health objectives translate into measures with an effect on trade. For example, WTO rules require non-discrimination in the application of trade measures. Discrimination may be particularly difficult to justify on health grounds, as it should not matter where unsafe

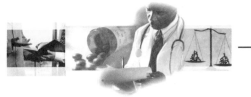

goods or services come from: for instance, meat containing a certain hazardous contaminant should be equally unwelcome irrespective of its origin. The Asbestos case illustrates another example of a health measure with an effect on trade (see section III, Box 10). In this case, there was a need to determine whether the measure was "necessary" to qualify for a general exception under Article XX(b). It was rather easy to determine that asbestos posed a serious health risk, but it was more difficult to decide whether the measures taken did not significantly favour French industry or whether "controlled use" as proposed by Canada might not offer the right level of health chosen by France. Through a process of "weighing and balancing" of different factors involved (such as the importance of the common interests or values protected by the measure or the efficacy of such measure in pursuing the policies aimed at) an import ban was ultimately found necessary to protect health.

284. Emphasizing and clarifying the scope that exists in WTO Agreements for conducting health-sensitive policies, and strengthening the capacity of national health authorities to contribute to policy coordination and to articulate "their" negotiating priorities may contribute to avoiding tensions. In this vein, many countries are increasing collaboration between trade and health to achieve national goals; Thailand and Canada are two such countries.[81] These national examples are followed by a discussion of how WHO and WTO are seeking improved cooperation at the international level.

(i) Thailand

285. The Thai Ministry of Health became aware of the importance of international trade law to health issues in the mid 1980s, when Thailand was placed on the US' Section 301 "trade-watch" list, because Thai law did not grant patents for pharmaceutical products. This was also the period when Thailand was engaged in Uruguay Round negotiations, and this led to discussions about the health implications of adding intellectual property rights protection to international trade agreements. Around the same period, trade and health groups in Thailand debated the desirability of opening up the tobacco market to foreign cigarette manufacturers. As a result of the need for a common government policy on these issues, the Health Ministry developed a strong, positive relationship with the Commerce Ministry's Department of Business Economics, which is responsible for all international trade agreements, including those in the WTO.

---

[81] Our thanks go to the Health Ministries of Thailand and Canada who contributed these case studies. It would be instructive to have more information on policy coordination processes between health and trade ministries in other countries that may have chosen different approaches to pursue policy coherence between trade and health.

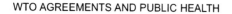

286. The Thai government's Foreign Trade Policy Committee, chaired by a Deputy Prime Minister, includes the Permanent Secretary for Health. This provides a high-level forum in which health interests can be considered in trade policy discussions. The Committee has several subcommittees addressing trade issues and the Permanent Secretary for Health sits on most of them, including those for TRIPS, GATS, and SPS/TBT. Also, many of the subcommittees have working groups in which other senior Ministry of Health staff participate. These same committees and working groups also address regional health-and-trade issues.

287. The Health Ministry has built up a network of health staff who understand trade issues and have the ability to advise trade officials. A Health Ministry focal point for trade issues has been designated within the Bureau of Health Policy and Planning, which coordinates health participation in trade issues. For each health-related trade issue, one of the Health Ministry department's serves as another focal point, e.g. the Division of Medical Registration, which controls all private hospitals and private medical personnel is the focal point for trade in services. For TRIPS, the focal point is the Food and Drug Administration, and for SPS and TBT, the focal point is the Department of Medical Science.

288. In 1998, the Ministry of Health established a Ministerial Commission on International Trade and Health, which brings together academic experts, civil society and the Ministry of Trade representatives to discuss key health-and-trade issues. One subcommittee has studied the effects of pipeline protection on the price of drugs. Another subcommittee has debated what the position of Thai delegates should be in the WTO or other international forums. For example, they debated Thailand's position for the June 2001 meeting of the WTO TRIPS Council's special discussion on TRIPS and access to drugs. Another project is studying the details of implementing parallel imports and compulsory licensing - who must be involved, which steps must be followed, and what the national patent law provides. On the General Agreement on Trade in Services (GATS), there is a project to study the implications of GATS on human resource development in Thailand. To further build national capacity to analyze the health implications of international trade, a special group has been supported to study these issues in the College of Public Health at Chulalongkorn University, sponsored by the Thailand Research Fund. Thailand's experience in health-and-trade collaboration indicates that top-level coordination contributes to ensuring that health interests are taken into account in trade policies.

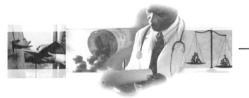

(ii) Canada

289. Collaboration between the Canadian health and trade ministries began in the early 1990s, prompted by negotiations with the United States and later Mexico on what became the North American Free Trade Agreement (NAFTA). Collaboration continued as Canada negotiated various bilateral trade agreements, the Uruguay Round of the WTO, and the Multilateral Agreement on Investment (where there was no agreement). Discussions included sanitary and phytosanitary measures, technical barriers to trade, intellectual property, investment, services, government procurement, and temporary entry of professionals.

290. Since 1999, the health department - called Health Canada - has taken a more strategic and coordinated approach to the interface with international trade issues to ensure early consideration of health policy concerns in trade discussions. This change was prompted by increasing recognition within the health ministry of the growing impact of international trade on health. This led to closer liaison and dialogue with trade officials and extensive participation by health ministry officials at all levels in the trade ministry's policy committees, working groups, and interdepartmental consultations. Trade officials also sought the participation of other departments to help prepare positions on current trade negotiations.

291. To forge a productive working relationship between the two ministries, Health Canada established a contact/focal point for trade officials to make it easier for trade officials to seek the views of the health ministry. The International Affairs Directorate assumed this role and set up a working group on international trade policy within Health Canada to bring together various health officials involved in health-and-trade issues (e.g., food safety, pharmaceuticals and patent protection, technical barriers, health services, health human resources, telehealth/telemedicine).

292. A better understanding of each other's perspectives and issues is aided by various interdepartmental mechanisms and processes set up by the trade ministry to address trade policy issues. Health officials' participation in these fora has helped them see how health-and-trade issues fit into the bigger picture. In addition, more informal dialogue and information sharing across government departments has proven invaluable.

293. The working relationship with the trade ministry has facilitated consultation on issues having health and trade dimensions. This includes, for example, trade disputes such as the asbestos case, trade negotiations (e.g., GATS, Free Trade Area of the Americas-FTAA), trade issues (e.g., TRIPS and essential medicines), trade communications (e.g., related to Canadian negotiating positions), private sector consultations (e.g., with health sector stakeholders on GATS), and WTO and NAFTA developments in general.

294. Health ministry influence on any particular trade position depends on several factors, including: the nature of the trade issue, how central the health policy question is to the issue, the importance of other domestic policy concerns, and existing positions (e.g. in trade agreements) on health and trade. Research evidence can be important, depending on the soundness and certainty of findings on the relationship between trade or trade agreements and health. Ultimately, trade negotiating positions are guided by overriding domestic policy priorities and objectives. Deciding which priorities take precedence requires health officials to explain clearly the national health priorities and objectives on which a trade position should be based.

C. INTERNATIONAL HEALTH-TRADE COORDINATION BETWEEN THE WHO AND WTO

295. At the international level, the WHO and the WTO are making efforts to co-ordinate their activities in several areas. At the highest political level, both organizations have addressed health-and-trade issues. At the technical level, the organizations recently held a workshop on differential pricing of drugs and the role of intellectual property rights.[82]

296. While the roles and objectives of the two organizations are distinct, there is potential for complementing each other's work. The issue of food safety is a good example of how this works on a day-to-day basis. The SPS Agreement encourages Members to base their food safety measures on international standards, guidelines and recommendations, where they exist. For food safety, the SPS Agreement explicitly refers to the standards, guidelines and recommendations established by the Codex (for which the WHO is a parent organisation). The usefulness of this link lies in the clarity it bestows on the distinct roles of the two organizations: on the one hand the evidence-based nature of WHO's scientific work and, on the other, the more legal trade-related

---

[82]. The final report can be found at: http://www.who.int/medicines/.

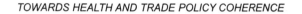
obligations under the WTO. In practice, this means that measures based on international standards, guidelines or recommendations developed by the Codex are presumed to be consistent with the SPS Agreement, and Members who base their measures on them can be confident of their compliance with WTO rules, and confident that consumers are being adequately protected.

297. Moreover, the link between the standard-setting work of the Codex and the scientific input from the WHO is important in that it lends some dynamics to the trade rules. While countries negotiate trade rules in the WTO, the WTO is not a scientific body and it does not develop standards. The WHO's active presence at SPS meetings has allowed WHO staff to provide advice on health matters relevant to trade. Examples are WHO's input on the risks of mad cow disease (BSE) to human health, and on the health effects of genetically-modified organisms in food. WHO representatives have also provided expert testimony to WTO dispute settlement panels, for example in the EC-Hormones case.

298. Aside from formal meetings, staff from the two organizations participate in regional or country-level meetings sponsored by one or both agencies for the purpose of providing technical assistance. For example, the WHO together with FAO provides technical assistance to countries to help them conform to SPS requirements by strengthening National Codex Committees, providing training in risk analysis, surveillance and control of food-borne diseases, and updating food legislation and improvement of food safety control systems. The WTO has frequently organised national or regional workshops on the SPS Agreement in close cooperation with Codex, the OIE and the secretariat of IPPC. In other contexts, the WHO has provided countries with technical advice on how to integrate public health perspectives into national patent legislation, and legally available options under the TRIPS agreement to promote equitable access to essential medicines. In September 2001, the WHO held a week-long training course for health and trade officials on the health implications of multilateral trade agreements, to which the WTO contributed.[83]

299. In addition to the SPS Committee, the WHO's official relationship with the WTO also includes observer status in the TBT and TRIPS Councils, and at the WTO Ministerial Meetings, though not in the General Council, for instance.[84] Observer status in relevant bodies increases the WHO's ability to identify mutually-supportive health and trade policies, and to help forestall potential conflicts. The WTO has observer status at the

---

[83.] More information on this course can be obtained directly from the WHO.

[84.] The issue of observer status is decided by WTO Member governments on a consensus basis.

WHO's annual meeting of the World Health Assembly. Also, WTO staff participate as observers in meetings of the Codex and in the deliberations on the Framework Convention on Tobacco Control.

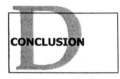

D. CONCLUSION

300. To make progress towards policy coherence, constructive engagement is critical on the key health-and-trade policy issues currently under consideration within the WTO, WHO and other international organizations. There are increasing opportunities for taking advantage of synergies between trade and health policies at the national and international level. At the international level, WTO and WHO meetings and negotiations represent important fora to examine the intersection of such policies. Some trade and health issues dealt with in WTO bodies and other international fora are shown in the box below (see Box 19).

301. Preparing policy decisions is not the sole province of government officials. On any specific issue the process involves several national players - ministries, specialized agencies, civil society, the private sector, and the public at large. Effective policy making depends on awareness, coordination and engagement of all those concerned. What follows are several actions which may contribute to policy coherence.

Box 19
Some trade and health issues in WTO bodies and other international fora

| TRIPS | • Review of the provisions of Article 27.3(b) |
| | • Intellectual property and access to medicines |

GATS	• Desirability and possible structure of an emergency safeguard mechanism
	• Domestic regulation (e.g. qualification, certification and licensing requirements)
	• Movements of natural persons

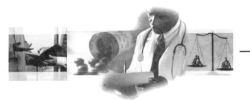

Box 19
Some trade and health issues in WTO bodies and other international fora (cont'd)

SPS and TBT	• Efficient participation of developing countries in standard-setting processes • Biotechnology • BSE • Antibiotic resistance
FCTC	• Negotiations on Framework Convention on Tobacco Control • Trade effects of potential provisions concerning international harmonization of taxes, packaging and labelling requirements, exemption of tobacco products from reduced tariffs under regional trade agreements, and advertising restrictions
IHR	• Revision of the International Health Regulations. • Consistency between WHO recommendations in "health emergencies of international concern" and SPS rules
Codex	• Codex food safety standards • Effective participation of developing countries in the Codex standard-setting processes (safety, quality and nutritional uses) • Safety standards and pre-market approval systems for foods derived from biotechnology (genetically modified foods)

(i) Addressing health issues in WTO rules

302. This document has highlighted ways in which WTO rules affect public health policy across a range of issues (infectious disease control, food safety, tobacco, environment, access to drugs, health services, food security and some emerging issues relevant to health such as biotechnology). All of these issues are addressed at regular meetings of the WTO. They may come up for discussion under a specific agenda item, as did the

issue regarding cholera in fish trade between Africa to Europe. Or a health issue may be the subject of focused discussions, as was the case with the TRIPS' Council meeting on patents and access to affordable medicines. It is useful for delegations attending these meetings to be aware of implicit health issues that may arise in the trade context. The participation of health officials when health issues are in focus can be helpful in this regard.

303. Aside from the work undertaken in the operational committees (agriculture, SPS, TBT etc.), the WTO Trade Policy Review Mechanisms (TPRM) may also provide a forum to discuss trade and health issues. The mandate of the TPRM suggests that a review of a Member's trade policy "takes place to the extent relevant, against the background of the wider ...development needs, policies and objectives of the member...". If health issues are viewed as a constraint on developmental objectives or trade policy implementation, there is an opportunity to raise them in the context of the review. Policy reviews could, in this manner, facilitate better interaction between government agencies responsible for trade policy. For example, it could be useful to outline health conditions in the TPRs, as part of the details provided on the human resources of the country under review (e.g., literacy, size, etc.). Secondly, health-and-trade issues could be germane to particular sections of the TPR reports dealing with health related topics, such as SPS, GATS and the TRIPS Agreement.

(ii) ... and trade issues in international health rules

304. Trade input into health policy making could also increase policy coherence. This requires the analysis of possible effects of proposed trade provisions in international health treaties and rules, and their consistency with the WTO agreements. This is similar to ongoing discussions of the consistency of trade provisions of MEAs with WTO rules, in the WTO Trade and Environment Committee (CTE) as well as in the related negotiations taking place in the CTE meeting in Special Sessions. "Trade impact assessment" is already being done informally through WTO monitoring of the on-going negotiations on the Framework Convention on Tobacco Control (FCTC). In this context, the WTO Secretariat provides information to clarify trade rules and attempts to draw attention to areas of potential conflict between WTO rules and provisions of the FCTC. Other examples for input from the trade side could be in the development of the WHO International Health Regulations and multilateral environmental agreements relevant to public health.

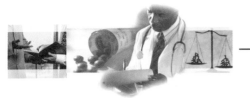

(iii) The need for evidence to inform policy

305. To monitor and evaluate the health impacts of existing WTO agreements and assess the potential health effects of proposed WTO rules and disciplines, there is a need for research and analysis. A current obstacle to analysis is the absence of systematic data collection, particularly in the area of trade in health services. Major data sources base statistics on trade in services only on modes 1 and 2 (cross-border provision and consumption abroad) and to a limited extent mode 4 (movement of natural persons), and often have only partial country coverage, depending on actual reporting practices, even in these areas. Commercial presence data are not covered by international statistics and there are no clear, agreed definitions of how the value of such trade would be measured. Existing national data relevant to these modes - for example on movement of consumers and providers, workers' remittances and direct investment - are not normally sufficiently disaggregated to separate out the components relating to the health sector, let alone to distinguish between, for example, movements by doctors and nurses, or direct investment in hospitals and other health-related services and facilities. There is an urgent need to improve data collection systems for a rigorous assessment of the extent, nature and geographical pattern of trade in health services (as defined by the GATS), and of the effects of services liberalization, including GATS commitments, on health and health systems.

(iv) Negotiation and reviews

306. Trade rules are negotiated by government officials often over several years. At WTO ministerial meetings (which take place at least once every two years) countries may decide on launching negotiations in new areas or deepening reform in other areas. At the Fourth WTO Ministerial Conference in Doha, Qatar, in November 2001, WTO Members decided on a future work programme of the WTO, the "Doha Development Agenda", which foresees negotiations in many areas (see Annex 1 for the Doha Ministerial Declaration). Before Doha, mandated negotiations have already been underway in agriculture and services, which also provide an opportunity for governments to address public health issues. Food security and health services are examples of health issues dealt with in this report which are relevant to these two areas. Furthermore, many WTO Agreements are regularly reviewed: the TRIPS Agreement is currently under review and the TBT Agreement is reviewed every three years. Governments may decide to involve health officials in domestic policy preparations to ensure that national health objectives are taken into account in any changes to the WTO agreements. They may also

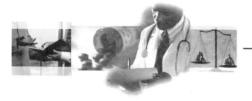

decide to include health officials on their international negotiating teams. The negotiations provide a crucial opportunity to address perceived imbalances, constraints or clarify provisions that are not sufficiently clear; they also provide an opportunity for amendments to be argued for and made, or even the creation of new agreements or understandings.

307. The importance of addressing concerns in the context of negotiations cannot be overstated. Negotiation in the WTO is a multilateral process, i.e. all Members of the Organization are involved and treated equally. While this makes it difficult and time-consuming to make progress on difficult and/or controversial issues, an eventual agreement can only be reached by consensus of all members. In case of disagreement on the meaning or the implications of a specific provision of a WTO agreement, individual countries can bring the matter to the Dispute Settlement Body. It would then be up to a panel, and possibly, the Appellate Body, to resolve the dispute.

(v) Accession

308. When a country applies for WTO membership, health and other officials have an additional opportunity to learn about the WTO and its agreements. It also provides an important avenue for health professionals in acceding countries to influence health-related trade policy. Accession is a negotiated process. Experience shows that the breadth and depth of the commitments, i.e. the number of sectors included and the levels of access bound, undertaken by acceding countries has increased in recent years.

(vi) Capacity-building

309. Policy coherence requires coordination across the areas of trade and health. This point has been emphasized throughout this whole report. In many developing countries, let alone least-developed countries, such capacity does not exist, or is very weak. Perhaps the greatest challenge in making trade a positive force for development is ensuring that the benefits accelerate development in the poorest countries and for the poorest people. The root of many health problems in developing countries is poverty. The Integrated Framework (IF) for Trade-Related Technical Assistance was set up to help LDCs become more integrated into the global economy.[85] During the reorganization of the IF in the summer of 2000, the six core agencies (IMF, ITC, UNCTAD, UNDP, World Bank and WTO) stressed that its objective was to ensure that trade policy is "articulated in a broad development context." The group emphasized that its advice and support

---

85. For more detail, see: www.ldcs.org.

should be closely linked to efforts by LDCs to develop national development strategies, either in the context of preparing Poverty Reduction Strategy Papers (PRSPs) for the World Bank and IMF, or under the UN Development Assistance Framework. WHO might work more closely with the IF to ensure that the trade-related advice offered by the international partners reflects health interests and objectives. In turn, work on these issues at the country level would inform policy-making at the international level in all of these organizations.

(vii) Two critical ingredients to policy coherence

310. Health and trade officials in all countries, along with representatives of civil society and the private sector, may use a wide array of fora and opportunities for achieving more coherence between policies. The resulting synergies would make a valuable contribution to more equitable and efficient human and economic development around the world. As already indicated above, there seem to be two critical ingredients, which significantly contribute to effective health-and-trade policy coordination.

311. The first is leadership. Key people in relevant ministries or international organizations must be knowledgeable about the issues of mutual concern and share information, including on upcoming policy decisions. Senior officials can set an example for collaboration by demonstrating their own commitment - in time, visibility, and resources - to cross-sectoral discussions and debates, including efforts to involve and inform civil society. Leadership is particularly important to avoid potential conflicts between hitherto not closely coordinated policy areas, such as health and trade.

312. Second, cross-sectoral institutions are important. Standing committees, task forces, working groups, or other bodies - whether at the national or international level that allow for regular contacts facilitate collaboration. In addition, government agencies could consult regularly with civil society, the private sector and academic experts to generate knowledge and public awareness of the issues, which in turn feed into the political decision-making process.

313. With these key ingredients, it is more likely that health and trade policies will interact in ways that are mutually supportive within the framework of global rules and institutions. The interface between health and trade becomes more critical in a fast-changing, more interconnected world. With the information and resources available today, policy synergies can be used to advance the common goal of sustainable human development for all peoples.

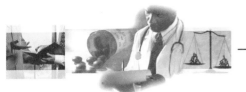

ANNEX

Other information resources on health and trade:

Further information on health and trade issues can be obtained from the sources listed below. While not exhaustive, this list provides a short-cut to different sources of information and points of view, nearly all of which can be accessed on-line. It is organized into six categories:

- Newsletters and Journals
- Intergovernmental Trade & Development Organizations
- UN/International Organizations with health-and-trade interests
- Non-governmental Organizations
- Health-and Trade Institutes - Academic and Independent
- Glossaries of Common Health and Trade Terms

NEWSLETTERS AND JOURNALS

ICTSD

The International Centre for Trade and Sustainable Development, an independent non-profit organization that aims to contribute to a better understanding of development and environmental concerns in the context of international trade, publishes two newsletters:

1.   BRIDGES Weekly Trade News Digest *http://www.ictsd.org/html/newsdigest.htm*
        A weekly e-mail newsletter on trade and sustainable development that offers a blend of original reporting and syntheses of trade news from other news media. Subscribe to receive e-mail versions.

2.   BRIDGES Between Trade and Sustainable Development
http://www.ictsd.org/html/arct_sd.htm.

        Monthly news and analysis on trade and sustainable development, plus periodic Latin American (in Spanish), African (in French) and German editions. Includes calendar of events, new publications and resources.

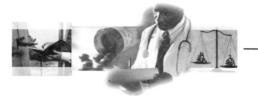

Inside US Trade   *http://www.insidetrade.com*
A weekly newsletter published by Inside Washington Publishers with in-depth coverage of US and international trade policy and WTO-related issues. Available to subscribers in on-line or print version. For subscription details contact iwp@sprintmail.com

———————————

World Trade Organization   *http://www.wto.org/english/res_e/focus_e/focus_e.htm*
The WTO publishes an electronic newsletter, FOCUS, 10 times a year in English, French and Spanish. Articles provide updates on key WTO activities and preview upcoming meetings. You can subscribe from any page on the WTO website by clicking on "Register" and choosing your area of interest.

———————————

Trade, Development and Economics Journals
http://www1.worldbank.org/wbiep/trade/TD_JOURNALS.html
Over two dozen journals dealing with trade and economics issues, including Journal of World Trade, Journal of Development Economics, Developing Economies Quarterly, are listed on the World Bank's Trade website. The site provides links to most of them and in many cases, you can perform on-line searches of the tables of contents and article for topics of interest.

———————————

Other journals that occasionally cover health-and-trade or health-and-globalization issues include:
Development, published by Society for International Development
http://www.sidint.org
Bulletin of the World Health Organization   *http://www.who.int/bulletin/*
          Lancet   *http://www.thelancet.com/journal*

———————————

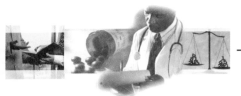

INTERGOVERNMENTAL TRADE AND DEVELOPMENT ORGANIZATIONS

World Trade Organization   *http://www.wto.org*

Rue de Lausanne 154

CH-1211 Geneva 21, Switzerland

Tel: (41-22) 739 51 11

Fax: (41-22) 731 42 06

email: enquiries@wto.org

The WTO's top level decision-making body is the Ministerial Conference which meets at least once every two years and is attended by Member governments' leading trade officials. WTO decisions are made by the entire membership, nearly always by consensus. WTO agreements must be ratified in all members' parliaments.

The General Council, which is usually attended by ambassadors and heads of delegation in Geneva, or officials sent from Members' capitals, meets several times a year in the Geneva headquarters. The General Council also meets as the Trade Policy Review Body and the Dispute Settlement Body.

At the next level, the Goods Council, Services Council and Intellectual Property (TRIPS) Council report to the General Council. The Goods Council has several committees, among them those on SPS and TBT. (Note: WHO currently has observer status in the TRIPS Council and the SPS and TBT Committees). Numerous specialized committees, working groups and working parties deal with the individual agreements and other areas such as the environment, development, membership applications and regional trade agreements, trade and investment, trade and competition policy, and transparency in government procurement.

The WTO Secretariat, based in Geneva, has around 550 staff and is headed by a Director-General. The Secretariat does not have the decision-making role common to other international agencies. Instead, its role is to provide technical support for the various councils and committees and the ministerial conferences, deliver technical assistance to developing countries, analyse world trade, and provide liaison with the public and media. The Secretariat also provides legal assistance in the dispute settlement process and advises governments wishing to become members of the WTO.

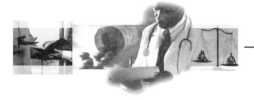

Technical Assistance and Training for Developing Countries. For an overview of WTO's TA, see: *http://www.wto.org/english/thewto_e/teccop_e/teccop_e.htm#guide*

The WTO organizes around 100 technical cooperation missions to developing countries annually. It holds on average three trade policy courses each year in Geneva for government officials. Regional seminars are held regularly, with a special emphasis on African countries. Training courses are also organized in Geneva for officials from countries in transition to market economies. The WTO has also set up reference centres in over 100 trade ministries and regional organizations in capitals of least-developed and developing countries, providing computers and Internet access to enable ministry officials to keep abreast of events in the WTO in Geneva through online access to the WTO's immense database of official documents and other material.

For a list of reference centres, see *http://www.wto.org/english/tratop_e/devel_e/listrc_e.doc*. LDCs currently are served by the Integrated Framework for Trade-Related Technical Assistance (IF). For further information, go to: *http://www.ldcs.org/*

The Trade Policy Review Mechanism provides a forum in which Member governments may openly discuss and provide an objective analysis of each others' trade policies, separate from the compliance-related and legal work of the WTO. Country Trade Policy reports provide an objective and independent review of the trade policies and practices of individual Members and portray an overall picture of the institutional interaction in trade policy formulation and implementation and the effect of policies on different sectors. In some cases, the reports serve as an input to trade policy formulation and several developing and least developed country Members have found the reviews valuable in identifying areas for potential technical assistance. See: *http://www.wto.org/english/tratop_e/tpr_e/tpr_e.htm*

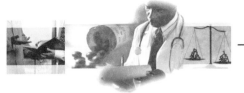

UN Conference on Trade and Development (UNCTAD) *http://www.unctad.org/*

Palais des Nations

1211 Geneva, Switzerland

Tel: (+41 22) 907 12 34

Fax: (+41 22) 907 00 43

E-mail: ers@unctad.org

UNCTAD is the focal point within the United Nations for development and interrelated issues in the areas of trade, finance, technology, investment and sustainable development. Its main goals are to maximize the trade, investment and development opportunities of developing countries. UNCTAD pursues its goals through research and policy analysis, intergovernmental deliberations, technical cooperation, and interaction with civil society and the business sector. UNCTAD conducts a number of meetings and produces publications to support countries in preparing for a new round of trade negotiations (see "Positive Agenda" site: *http://www.unctad.org/en/posagen/index.htm*).

UNCTAD has sponsored several expert meetings on health and trade issues, including one with WHO in 1998 on International Trade in Health Services (see UNCTAD/ITCD/TSB/5 or WHO/TFHE/98.1: International Trade in Health Services: A Development Perspective, available at: http://www.unctad.org/en/pub/poitcdtsbd5.en.htm. Recently, UNCTAD sponsored a meeting, in conjunction with WIPO and the Convention on Biological Diversity, to examine systems for protecting traditional knowledge, including traditional medicine knowledge and practices (see papers at: http://www.unctad.org/en/special/c1em13do.htm. UNCTAD also prepared a study on International Trade in Genetically Modified Organisms and Multilateral Negotiations: A New Dilemma for Developing Countries in July 2000 (UNCTAD/DITC/TNCD/1, unedited version).

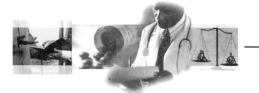
International Trade Centre (ITC)   *http://www.intracen.org*

Palais des Nations

1211 Geneva 10, Switzerland

Tel: (+41 22) 730 01 11

Fax: (+41 22) 733 44 39

E-mail: itcreg@intracen.org

The International Trade Centre (ITC) based in Geneva is the focal point in the United Nations system for technical cooperation with developing countries in trade promotion - both export and import operations. ITC is operated jointly with WTO and UNCTAD, and is an executing agency of UNDP-financed projects in developing countries related to trade promotion. ITC conducted a study on the implications of the multilateral trade agreements for international trade in medical devices (ITC/280/2D/99-III-TO). In conjunction with WHO, ITC's Market News Service issues a monthly report on Pharmaceutical Starting Materials/Essential Drugs, giving up-to-date indicative prices and relevant commercial data trends on 206 pharmaceutical Starting Materials used in the manufacturing of essential drugs (available on a subscription basis). ITC plans to publish a handbook on tourism and health services.

Regional Trading Organizations

For links to the major regional trading organizations, e.g. NAFTA, Mercosur, ASEAN, European Union, etc., see: *http://www1.worldbank.org/wbiep/trade/TD_REG_ORG.html*.

The European Commission's Trade Directorate has set up several civil society issue groups, one of which is health (*http://europa.eu.int/comm/trade/2000_round/issuegr.htm*). For information on EU trade policy developments, see: *http://europa.eu.int/comm/trade/*.

In addition, some regional inter-governmental organizations provide advice and information on trade-related issues. For example, the Organization of American States (OAS) Trade Unit assists the 34 OAS member countries with matters related to trade and economic integration in the Western Hemisphere and, in particular, with their efforts to establish a Free Trade Area of the Americas. Go to: *http://www.oas.org/* and click on "Trade and Integration" at the top of the website.

World Bank   *http://www.worldbank.org*

1818 H Street, NW

Washington, DC 20433, USA

Tel: 01-202-477-1234

Fax: 01-202-477-6391

The World Bank operates a comprehensive "International Trade and Development" website: *http://www1.worldbank.org/wbiep/trade/*. It serves "as a research, training and outreach tool for people interested in trade policy and developing countries. Particular emphasis is placed on the new trade agenda associated with the upcoming round of WTO negotiations. In addition to the capacity-building activities of the World Bank Institute and the World Bank's Research Group, it provides information on complementary programs through the Integrated Framework for Trade-Related Technical Assistance to Least Developed Countries (see above under WTO) and the joint World Bank-WTO website (see below).

The site offers distance learning courses and provides an extensive set of information (including data and databases) on various trade topics, including services, intellectual property rights and standards which may be of interest to a health audience. For example, the Standards site, contains many papers and resources providing insight into the effect of environmental, health, and safety requirements on producers of goods, services, and agricultural products. The site also has papers in Spanish, Russian and Chinese.

The Trade and Development Centre (*http://www.itd.org/*). The World Bank's Economic Development Institute runs a joint venture with the World Trade Organization called Information Technologies for Development (ITD). Its website serves "anyone interested in social and economic development and how these are related to trade. It offers information, analysis and comment on these issues and an opportunity to exchange views." Included are interactive guides and training courses on trade policy and interesting case studies from Africa and India on trade-and-health topics; one case describes the failed attempt in the US to patent turmeric for its healing properties.

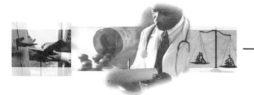

UN/INTERGOVERNMENTAL ORGANIZATIONS WITH HEALTH-AND-TRADE INTERESTS

World Health Organization (WHO)   *http://www.who.int/*

Avenue Appia 20

1211 Geneva 27, Switzerland

Tel: (+41 22) 791 2111

Fax: (+41 22) 791 3111

WHO conducts a variety of trade-and-health activities in each of its core functions:

(1) Articulating evidence-based policy and advocacy positions, e.g. on global trade rules that affect health; (2) managing information and conducting or stimulating research and development, e.g. on the risks to health from trade of various kinds; (3) providing technical advice and policy support to Member States, e.g. on implementing WTO agreements in ways that maximize health; (4) negotiating and sustaining national and global partnerships, e.g. to achieve coherence in national or global health-and-trade policies; (5) setting and promoting international norms and standards, e.g. to assure the quality, efficacy and safety of pharmaceuticals, biological substances, food, animal products, and pesticides that are internationally traded; and (6) testing or stimulating the development of new technologies, tools and guidelines for health protection and improvement. For further information, publications, and technical assistance on health-and-trade issues, follow links or send requests to the following departments:

General Trade Issues: Department of Health in Sustainable Development (website under construction, contact dragern@who.int with questions)

Pharmaceuticals and Patent Issues/TRIPS: *http://www.who.int/medicines/*

Food standards, food safety and trade: *http://www.who.int/fsf/*

International Health Regulations & SPS: *http://www.who.int/emc/IHR/int_regs.html*

Health Services and GATS: *http://www.who.int/health-services-delivery/trade/index.htm*

(website under construction, contact thompsona@who.int with questions)

Tobacco Control and Trade Issues: *http://tobacco.who.int/*

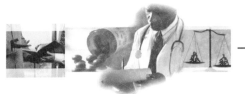

Some of WHO's six regional headquarters also have publications and activities to address health-and-trade issues. To contact them, follow the links at: *http://www.who.int/regions/*. From the WHO regional office websites, you can also access WHO's more than 100 country offices.

UN Food and Agriculture Organization (FAO)   *http://www.fao.org/*
Viale delle Terme di Caracalla
00100 Rome, Italy
Tel: +39(06)5705.1
Fax: +39(06)5705.4593

Through their joint sponsorship with WHO of the Codex Alimentarius Commission ("Codex") FAO sets and promotes food safety standards, guidelines and other recommendations for internationally traded foods. The Codex website is *http://www.codex-alimentarius.net/*. The Food and Nutrition Division offers information on biotechnology and food at: *http://www.fao.org/waicent/faoinfo/economic/ESN/gm/biotec-e.htm*. In 1999, FAO co-sponsored with WHO and WTO a conference on International Food Trade Beyond 2000, to review and assess the implementation of Codex work in the context of the Uruguay Round trade agreements. See report at:
http://www.fao.org/WAICENT/FAOINFO/ECONOMIC/ESN/austral/austra-e.htm

FAO provides technical assistance to provide member countries in building their capacity to deal with trade-related food safety and security issues, both in the implementation of Uruguay Round Agreements and preparing developing countries for upcoming multilateral trade negotiations. See information at: *http://www.fao.org/ur/*. *The* Agricultural Policy Support Service (TCAS) at FAO runs a program on "Policies for Agricultural Trade" *(http://www.fao.org/tc/tca/wlcm.htm)* which provides information and assistance to countries on the economic implications of international and regional trade agreements. In addition, to assist countries in multilateral trade negotiations on agriculture, FAO runs a world-wide training programme; see
http://www.fao.org/ur/umbrella.htm) for more information.

Office International des Epizooties (OIE)   *http://www.oie.int*

12, rue de Prony, 75017 Paris, France

Tel: 33 - (0)1 44 15 18 88

Fax: 33 - (0)1 42 67 09 87

Website: www.oie.int

E-mail: oie@oie.int

Founded in 1924, the OIE is an intergovernmental organization with 158 members. Its main aims are to guarantee the transparency of animal disease status world-wide, collect, analyze and disseminate veterinary scientific information, provide expertise and promote international solidarity for the control of animal diseases; and guarantee the sanitary safety of world trade by developing sanitary rules for international trade in animals and animal products. The Office is placed under the authority and control of an International Committee consisting of Delegates designated by the Governments of Member Countries. The day-to-day operation of the OIE is managed by a Central Bureau situated in Paris, placed under the responsibility of a Director General elected by the International Committee. The Central Bureau implements the resolutions passed by the International Committee and developed with the support of elected Commissions.

Organization for Economic Cooperation & Development (OECD) *http://www.oecd.org/*

2, rue André Pascal

F-75775 Paris Cedex 16, France

Tel.: +33-1-45-24-8200

OECD's Trade Committee has not taken up trade-and-health related activities, though there have been some proposals to initiate activity in health-care services (e.g. by EC and some EU Member States). Biotechnology-related work at OECD is undertaken in several different tracks (see *http://www.oecd.org/ehs/icgb/*): e.g. food safety, agriculture, intellectual property rights, and human health. OECD's main focus is on the international harmonization of regulatory oversight in biotechnology and to ensure that environmental health and safety aspects are properly evaluated while avoiding non-tariff trade barriers to biotechnology products. OECD has taken an active role in the food safety and quality debate, in particular the scientific and health aspects of genetically modified (GM) foods. The report on "Food Safety and Quality: Trade Considerations" published in November 1999 examines trade conflicts arising from food safety and quality issues, summarizes the key international agreements, and reviews the potential contributions of economic analysis to conflict resolution.

South Centre *http://www.southcentre.org/*

Case Postale 228

1211 Geneva 19, Switzerland

Tel: (41 22) 791 80 50

Fax: (41 22) 798 85 31

Created in 1995, the South Centre is an intergovernmental body of developing countries. Currently 46 countries are members, but the Centre works for the benefit of the South as a whole. They assist in developing points of view of the South on major policy issues, and help to generate ideas and action-oriented proposals for governments, intergovernmental organizations, NGOs and others. They conduct workshops and publish many trade-related publications and documents, including a quarterly newsletter, South Letter, which can be viewed on-line at: *http://www.southcentre.org/southletter/index.htm*, and a fortnightly newsletter, called South Bulletin. One of their most recent reports is Integrating Public Health Concerns Into Patent Legislation In Developing Countries by Carlos Correa, of the University of Buenos Aires, Argentina; it can be downloaded at: *http://www.southcentre.org/publications/publichealth/toc.htm*

UN Development Program (UNDP)   *http://www.undp.org/*

One United Nations Plaza

New York, NY 10017, USA

Tel: +1-212.906-5302

Fax: +1-212-906-5364

E-mail: aboutundp@undp.org

UNDP is a core member of the Integrated Framework for Trade-Related Technical Assistance. Through its country offices, it works with the other core members (WTO, UNCTAD, ITC, IMF, and the World Bank) in assisting countries to integrate trade policy within broader poverty reduction strategies at the national level. The UN Development Fund for Women (UNIFEM), based at UNDP, has a Program on Women and International Trade, which maintains a website (*http://www.undp.org/unifem/trade/home.htm*) that brings together information on "trade issues and their gender-differentiated impact on women." UNIFEM sponsors training and workshops and publishes documents.

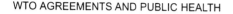

World Intellectual Property Organization (WIPO)   *http://www.wipo.org/*

P.O. Box 18

CH-1211 Geneva 20, Switzerland

Tel: 41 22 338 91 11

Fax: 41 22 733 54 28

E-mail: wipo.mail@wipo.int

WIPO, one of 16 specialized UN agencies with 175 Member States, administers 21 international treaties dealing with different aspects of intellectual property protection. Details of these treaties can be found at: http://www.wipo.org/treaties/index.html can be divided into three general groups: (1) treaties that define internationally agreed basic standards of intellectual property protection in each country, e.g. the Paris, Berne, and Rome Conventions; (2) registration treaties, which ensures that one international registration or filing will have effect in any of the relevant signatory States, and (3) classification treaties, which create classification systems that organize information concerning inventions, trademarks and industrial designs into indexed, manageable structures for easy retrieval. WIPO has projects or provides technical assistance in the area of systems for protecting traditional medicine knowledge and practice, pharmaceutical-intellectual property rights issues and IPR issues in health-related electronic commerce (e.g. pharmaceuticals, trademarks, counterfeits, and privacy-issues).

NON-GOVERNMENTAL ORGANIZATIONS

Consumers International (CI) *www.consumersinternational.org.*

24 Highbury Crescent

London, N5 1RX, United Kingdom

Tel: +44 171 226 6663

Fax: +44 171 354 0607

E-mail: consint@consint.org

Consumers International (CI) is an independent, non-profit organization that supports, links and represents consumer groups and agencies all over the world. It has a membership of more than 260 organizations in almost 120 countries and maintains several regional offices around the world. It defends the rights of all consumers, including poor, marginalized and disadvantaged people, by campaigning at the international level for policies which respect consumer concerns. Among its current campaigns are: (1) Trade and Economics, to ensure that international trade agreements benefit consumers by lobbying at the WTO and other global and regional organizations, and researching trade-related issues such as agricultural liberalization, intellectual property rights, competition policy and investment policy; (2) Health, to promote the rational use of essential drugs, universal high quality health care services, and patients' rights, and (3) Food and Sustainable Agriculture, to improve nutrition and food standards by involvement in the Codex Alimentarius Commission and campaigning on GMO and food security issues. A publications catalogue, briefing papers, press releases and updates about campaigns are included on its website.

Consumers International also serves as the Secretariat for the Trans Atlantic Consumer Dialogue (within CI's Programmes for Developed Economies). The Transatlantic Consumer Dialogue (http://www.tacd.org/) is a forum of US and EU consumer organizations which develops and agrees joint consumer policy recommendations to the US government and European Union to promote consumer interest in EU and US policy making. TACD addresses issues of high priority to consumer organizations such as trade in services, access to medicines, GM foods, private data protection and transparency in government.

Consumer Project on Technology (CPT)   *http://www.cptech.org*

P.O. Box 19367

Washington, DC 20036, USA

Tel: +1.202.387.8030

Fax: +1.202.234.5176

By email, for intellectual property and health care:

James Love : love@cptech.org   or

Thiru Balasubramaniam : thiru@cptech.org

The Consumer Project on Technology is a non-profit, consumer organization started by Ralph Nader in 1995. Currently CPT is focusing on intellectual property rights and health care, electronic commerce (very broadly defined) and competition policy. Its website has a large number of documents, articles, and correspondence among key actors involved in these issues. For example, its web page on health care, regional trade agreements and intellectual property rights, has links to IP activities in FTAA, NAFTA & APEC and other regional trade groups: (*http://www.cptech.org/ip/health/trade/*). The country disputes page has documentation on IP-pharmaceutical issues in 12 countries *http://www.cptech.org/ip/health/country/*.

European Public Health Alliance (EPHA)   *http://www.epha.org/*
33 rue de Pascale
1040 Brussels, Belgium
Tel: +32 2 230 30 56
E-mail: epha@epha.org

EPHA represents over 70 non-governmental and other not-for-profit organizations working in support of health in Europe. EPHA issues a bi-monthly magazine on health policy in the EU and Europe - the European Public Health Update, to which non-members can subscribe, available in English, French and German. EPHA organized a meeting in April 2000 on how WTO agreements and EU policies may affect health policies, both in developing countries and European countries. Some of the papers presented at that meeting are available at: *http://www.epha.org/public/campaigns/wto.htm*

Health Action International   *http://www.haiweb.org/*
c/o: HAI Europe
Jacob van Lennepkade 334-T
1053 NJ Amsterdam, The Netherlands
Tel: (+31-20) 683 3684
Fax: (+31-20) 685 5002
E-mail: hai@hai.antenna.nl

HAI is a non-profit, global network of more than 150 health, development, consumer and other public interest groups in more than 70 countries working for a more rational use of medicinal drugs. In addition to the European office, HAI has regional offices for

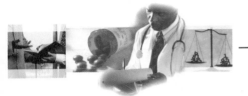

Latin America (based in Peru) and Asia and the Pacific Region (based in Malaysia). HAI is currently running advocacy campaigns on Increasing Access to Essential Drugs in a Globalised Economy and Compulsory Licensing of Medicines.

International Centre for Trade and Sustainable Development *http://www.ictsd.org/*

13 Chemin des Anémones

1219 Châtelaine, Geneva, Switzerland

Tel: (41-22) 731-5734

Fax: (41-22) 917-8093

E-mail: ictsd@ictsd.ch

Established in September 1996, ICTSD contributes to a better understanding of development and environment concerns in the context of international trade. As an independent non-profit and non-governmental organization, ICTSD engages a broad range of actors in dialogue about trade and sustainable development. With a wide network of partners, ICTSD provides reporting services on international trade and sustainable development. In addition to its weekly and monthly newsletters (see p. 1 of this Annex), it publishes in-depth analyses of specific issues connected to the world trading system. The website has a comprehensive set of background briefs on issues including trade issues/rules, trade developments, biotechnology and biosafety, health, environment, women's rights and gender issues, indigenous knowledge, intellectual property rights and human rights.

International Organization for Standardization (ISO)   *http://www.iso.ch/*

1, rue de Varembé

Case postale 56

CH-1211 Geneva 20, Switzerland

Tel: + 41 22 749 01 11

Fax: + 41 22 733 34 30

E-mail: central@iso.ch

One of ISO's best-known standards, the ISO 9000, provides a framework for quality management and quality assurance that is used by businesses throughout the world. The

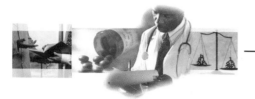

standards are now being revised - see http://www.iso.ch/9000e/revisionstoc.htm for updates on this revision process. Within the health field, ISO has developed standards for mechanical contraceptives (condoms, IUDs and rubber diaphragms), certain medical devices or surgical instruments, and lab glassware among other things. Recently, ISO developed eco-labelling standards (ISO 14020 and ISO 14024).

MEDACT   *http://www.medact.org/*

601 Holloway Road

London, N194DJ, UK

Tel: 020 7272 2020

Fax: 020 7281 5757

E-mail: info@medact.org

Medact is an organization of health professionals challenging social and environmental barriers to health worldwide. It highlights the health impacts of violent conflict, poverty and environmental degradation, and works to eradicate them. Medact has a report on "The World Trade Organization: Implications for Health Policy", available on its website.

Médicins sans Frontières (MSF)   *http://www.msf.org/*

MSF International Office:

Rue de la Tourelle, 39$

Brussels, Belgium, 1040

Tel: +32-2-280-1881

Fax: +32-2-280-0173

MSF is an independent humanitarian medical aid agency committed to providing medical aid wherever it is needed and raising awareness of the plight of the people it helps. MSF has offices in 19 countries, and operations in 84. The Campaign for Access to Essential Medicines was created to mobilize support for improved access to essential medicines. One of the campaign's three pillars involves health exceptions to trade agreements (mostly TRIPS). For more information, see: *http://www.accessmed.msf.org/* which has links to numerous documents and articles from around the world.

HEALTH-AND-TRADE INSTITUTES - ACADEMIC AND INDEPENDENT

Chulalongkorn University Social Research Institute (CUSRI) *http://focusweb.org/*

Wisit Prachuabmoh Building

Chulalongkorn University

Bangkok 10330 Thailand

Tel: (66 2) 218 7363

Fax: (66 2) 255 9976

E-mail: admin@focusweb.org

CUSRI runs Focus on the Global South, an autonomous programme of "progressive development policy research and practice" dedicated to regional and global policy analysis, micro-macro linking and advocacy work. It publishes Focus-on-Trade, a regular electronic bulletin (in English and Spanish) providing updates and analysis on regional and global trade and finance.

London School of Hygiene and Tropical Medicine

http://www.lshtm.ac.uk/centres/cgech/

Centre on Globalisation, Environmental Change & Health

Keppel St

London WC1E 7HT, United Kingdom

Tel: +44 (0) 207 612 7825

Fax: +44 (0) 207 580 6897

E-mail: cgech@LSHTM.ac.uk

Conducts cross-disciplinary research on globalization, environmental change and health. The website describes current research, lists recent publications and previews coming events.

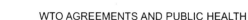

Globalisation and Social Policy Programme (GASPP)

http://www.stakes.fi/gaspp/

C/o: STAKES (National Research and Development Centre for Welfare and Health)

PO Box 220

FIN-00531, Helsinki,

Finland

Tel: +358 9 39 671

Fax: +358 761 307

GASPP is a five-year (1997-2002) research, advisory, education and public information programme based jointly at STAKES (National Research and Development Centre for Welfare and Health) based in Helsinki, Finland and the Centre for Research on Globalisation and Social Policy, Department of Sociological Studies, University of Sheffield, England. GASSP conducts research, provides policy advice, organizes conferences and seminars and publishes a number of books and papers (and a journal starting in 2001). GASSP currently has projects on: (1) the implications of the WTO and international trade agreements for health and social policies, and (2) the health implications of other EU policies.

Harvard University, Center for International Development

The Global Trade Negotiations Home Page *http://www.cid.harvard.edu/cidtrade/* is a resource for those interested in analytical information on the multitude of issues, debates, government positions, and organizations that surround international trade policy. It has a large collection of research papers and articles, links to other websites, as well as contact information for additional sources. The site allows you to navigate the Internet to find information on global trade policy and negotiations. Resources and links are organized by: Actors (National Governments, NGOs, International Organizations) and Trade Issue (SPS/TBT, electronic commerce, intellectual property and services, among many others).

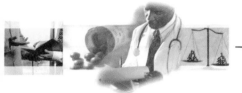

Institute of Development Studies (IDS)   *http://nt1.ids.ac.uk/eldis/*

University of Sussex

Brighton,

United Kingdom

Tel: +44 1273 877330

Fax: +44 1273 621202

E-mail: eldis@ids.ac.uk

IDS operates ELDIS, an Internet-based "Gateway to Information Sources on Development and the Environment". It provides descriptions and links to a wide variety of information sources, including online documents, organization's WWW sites, databases, library catalogues, bibliographies, and e-mail discussion lists, research project information, map and newspaper collections. It also describes available databases, CD-ROMs, etc. ELDIS has a special site devoted to international trade issues, complete with short background papers and links to many other international and research institutions, and statistical sources: *http://nt1.ids.ac.uk/eldis/trade/trade.htm*. ELDIS maintains a similar site devoted to international health issues, at:

http://nt1.ids.ac.uk/eldis/health/health.htm

Links to other trade-related institutes can be found at:

http://www1.worldbank.org/wbiep/trade/TD_INSTITUTIONS.html

Links to institutes or organizations that study and research general globalization issues:

http://www.globalpolicy.org/globaliz/websites.htm

GLOSSARIES OF COMMON HEALTH AND TRADE TERMS

WTO Glossary of Terms: An informal guide to 'WTO speak'

http://www.wto.org/english/thewto_e/minist_e/min01_e/brief_e/brief22_e.htm

Prepared for the Fourth WTO Ministerial Conference in November 2001. It is an online abridged version of the WTO Trilingual Glossary, "an immense vocabulary of trade"

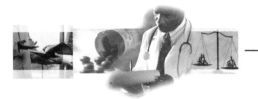

in English, French and Spanish. Many entries contain a reference to relevant sources and include acronyms, definitions, explanatory notes and other useful information. To order the Trilingual Glossary, order from the WTO on-line bookshop,
e-mail: publications@wto.org or go to: *http://www.wto.org/english/res_e/booksp_e/book-sp_e.htm*

Health-Related Terminology in Cyberspace http://www.who.int/terminology/ter/dic-fair.html
WHO maintains a list of medical dictionaries and glossaries, along with links to their websites. In addition to links to general medicine dictionaries, it has 20 specialized categories from AIDS to Tropical Medicine. WHO also has a terminology guide to the World Health Report 2000 on Health Systems:
http://www.who.int/terminology/ter/TERWB-WHR2000.htm, with translations into French, Spanish, Russian, Chinese and Arabic.

The ABCs of Trade Liberalization
UNIFEM's trade site has a directory of terms and acronyms in the trade arena, with links to many related websites. See *http://www.undp.org/unifem/trade/abchome.htm*.

The Terms of Trade and Other Wonders: Deardorff's Glossary of International Economics. *http://www-personal.umich.edu/~alandear/glossary/*

Includes definitions, links to definitions, and wherever appropriate links to other sites and documents that may provide additional information. "This glossary will eventually attempt to cover all of the terms and concepts from international economics, including both international trade and international finance, at least at the introductory level." Because the author's specialty is international trade, coverage in that area is more thorough.

Dictionary of Trade Policy Terms, Walter Goode, Centre for International Economic Studies, University of Adelaide

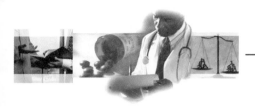

Glossary of trade terms, expressions and history of the multilateral trading system since 1947. This book is aimed at non-specialists using trade policy terms on a daily basis. The dictionary is available in English and can be ordered at *http://www.adelaide.edu.au/cies/orderform.htm.*